Shelley Bovey is a writer ~~~~~~~~~~~~~~~~~~~~~~~~~~~~~
prefers radio to television bec~~~~~~~~~~~~~~~~~~~~~~~~~~~~~
say is more important than hov~~~~~~~~~~~~~~~ contributor
to the *Guardian*, the *Independent* and several magazines, and is
the author of three books, including *The Forbidden Body: Why
Being Fat Is Not A Sin*. The mother of three grown-up
children, she lives in Somerset with her husband and a great
many animals.

Sizeable Reflections

Big Women
Living Full Lives

**Shelley Bovey,
editor**

First published by The Women's Press Ltd, 2000
A member of the Namara Group
34 Great Sutton Street, London EC1V 0LQ

Collection copyright © Shelley Bovey 2000

The copyright in each of the pieces in this collection remains with
the original copyright holder.

Cover illustration: The Bather, called "Baigneuse Valpincon", 1808
by Jean Auguste Dominique Ingres (1780–1867)
Louvre, Paris, France/Bridgeman Art Library

'How We Met: Dawn French and Helen Teague'
by Anthi Charalambous first appeared in the *Independent on Sunday*,
14 February 1999.

The right of Shelley Bovey and the contributors to be identified as
the joint authors of this work has been asserted by them in
accordance with the Copyright, Designs and Patents Act 1988.

British Library Cataloguing-in-Publication Data
A catalogue record for this book is available from the British Library.

This book is sold subject to the condition that it shall not, by way of
trade or otherwise, be lent, re-sold, hired out, or otherwise circulated
without the Publisher's prior consent in any form of binding or cover
other than that in which it is published and without a similar
condition including this condition being imposed on the subsequent
purchaser.

ISBN 0 7043 4587 0

Typeset in Bembo 11/13 pt by FSH Ltd, London
Printed and bound in Great Britain by Cox & Wyman Ltd, Reading,
Berkshire

for Jill
with love

Acknowledgements

My thanks to all the women who have contributed to this book and who, in doing so, have become friends.

And to Jill Welbourne for the title: Sizeable Reflections.

Contents

Introduction

This book is a celebration, a coming together of 24 successful, powerful women whose lives are testimony to the fact that being fat does not mean living beyond the pale. Not so very long ago, the only place you were likely to find a gathering of large women was at a slimming club and they certainly weren't there to celebrate, unless, of course, they had lost weight. As recently as ten years ago, women who were deemed overweight by society's moral, medical and aesthetic yardstick lived and moved in isolation. Ostracism and marginalisation make for loneliness. Fat people, fat women especially, often put their lives on hold, waiting for the time when they could perceive themselves as acceptable in their own and others' eyes.

This was a terrible waste of life but such is the strength of social persecution that many fat people set their sights at the lowest possible level because they had been told that is where they belonged. And too often, when they summoned the courage to prove otherwise, they were met with closed doors and painful rejections. It is still a fact that many fat people are refused college admission and are turned down for jobs and medical procedures for no other reason than that they are fat. Such is the superficiality of our culture that looks are paramount and appearance is all. One phrase remains indelibly in my mind as a brutal, though honest, summing up of the prevailing ethos: one woman applying for a health visitor's post was told, 'We've got so many applicants we don't need a fat one.' No other group in society is discriminated against so blatantly; it's always 'open season' on the overweight.

Most of the women who tell their stories here have known the pain of not belonging, of being told in a myriad different ways that they were not good enough because of their size. Some of them still feel something of that pain but it does not predominate. Their size is part of them but it does not define them; they have not in any way been defeated by their weight. And because of that, these essays are a triumph.

When I commissioned the pieces I asked the authors to make them as personal as they wanted. I wanted readers to go with these women on the journeys they had made to self-acceptance and beyond. That phrase, 'journeys to self-acceptance', can sound a little worthy, straight out of the self-help books, but there is no flavour of that in these stories. They are funny; they are fierce; they are moving, courageous and entertaining. Some of them are raw, some are bursting with confidence. None is self-deprecating. These are women who know that society has got it wrong. They have nothing to apologise for and nothing to hide.

Many different aspects of life as a fat woman are illustrated here. Jenni Murray and Kathryn Szrodecki demonstrate that contrary to popular myth, you can be fat and joyfully fit, while Betty Woods and Ali Jacques have made fatness into an artform – literally – with their photography and image-making. Lee Kennedy, the brilliant cartoonist, has sketched for us with a wry, mordant wit which is searingly perceptive and novelist Susan Stinson paints her story with rich almost edible poetry and prose.

Angela Kennedy takes a look at the not-so-positive role of the fat woman in contemporary film and Stephanie Jones sounds a warning about the equation that fat and black means acceptability. Former Australian actress, Maggie Millar, describes how the 'Body Police' made her profession in that country intolerable – while Miriam Margolyes and Jo Brand have managed to turn their size to their advantages as performers, and the results are richly humorous.

Sally E. Smith, Diana Pollard and Liz Swinden talk about

the size-acceptance movement and how we can change things if self-belief is strong enough. And Janice Bhend, the first British journalist to write about plus-size fashions, describes how she fulfilled a lifelong dream and launched a 'glossy' magazine for big women. Fulfilling a dream is something that occurs as a motif in many of these essays – women who were told that they would make nothing of their lives because they were fat rose to the top, like cream.

What stands out most in all these accounts is a sense of pride. Not the 'proud to be fat' claim which, for me, resonates with positive discrimination – but pride in achievement and in having a full, undamaged sense of self.

I hope that anyone feeling less than confident about their shape in our thin-worshipping society will be encouraged by these stories. They demonstrate that happiness and success are attainable at any size

Shelley Bovey
Somerset
January 2000

Fit to be Fat

Jenni Murray

It ranks, I have to confess, in the personal canon of 'most embarrassing moments'. Right up there with the kilt that fell about my knees during a recitation of *The Christmas Tree* at the Elsecar Music Festival circa 1954, and with discovering the obstetrician set to do the embroidery after the birth of my first child was a close family friend who fancied himself a better comedian than surgeon (don't even ask, but I have since led a relatively normal life!). This though, that first moment of exposure in a changing room, was a different kind of nightmare. This was Wilhelmina set free in a shatteringly shimmering shoal of shrimp or – as my children had so delicately put it – 'you look like a beached whale, Mum'. Which was where the killer instinct had kicked in. I had decided it was either infanticide or the gym.

I chose the latter, as a more socially acceptable option, and because I happened to notice while visiting the local off-licence (it was a 'bottle of fizzy wine and several packets of Kettle Chips' night – depressing) that a new 'American Style Fitness Centre' had opened just around the corner and was offering half price membership. For someone who normally takes a taxi to go to the end of the street, it seemed one hell of a walk – but, never one to resist what appears to be a bargain, I tottered off to their reception, made my enquiries, salivated over the sauna and Jacuzzi, pretended the cross trainers and weight machines weren't for the likes of me and signed on the dotted line.

There is, of course, I argued to myself on the way home, no more pointless activity than getting fit – sitting on a bike or walking a treadmill to nowhere is a criminal waste of human energy. It amazes me that no enterprising young blood has yet designed a method of attaching every gym in the land to the national grid. But good mean Yorkshire woman that I am, having handed over the hard cash, I couldn't bring myself to object on political or environmental grounds to turning up for my induction the following day. So there I was in a pair of extra large Donna Karan cycle shorts, the baggiest T-shirt Evans could provide, and an enormous sports bra from M&S, which those two lovely children of mine suggested might make a good hammock if stretched between two trees.

One look in the mirror (of which there are always millions in such changing rooms) and there indeed was the whale Wilhelmina surrounded by the lycra clad, glowing pink shrimps. It was an 'Oh God, open up the ground and let this ample form fall through' moment. But as usual, She wasn't listening — a bit like me when I first read Susie Orbach's *Fat is a Feminist Issue*. Listen to your appetite, she writes, and when you aren't hungry any more, just stop. It is the one subject on which I appear to be profoundly deaf. I digress.

Jason was allocated to me as my personal inductor. He appeared surprisingly unalarmed at my obvious lack of condition — he'd obviously seen it all before. We filled out a form about my general state of health, which unaccountably my doctor had informed me was really rather good. I was spared the humiliation of being weighed. (One lesson I did manage to pick up from Susie Orbach, far too dispiriting. Never diet, never weigh yourself.) Nor did I have to endure any humiliating measuring of body fat. 'No,' said Jason, 'the best thing is just to get started right away — just give me an idea of your objectives.'

I resisted the strong temptation to tell him my main objective was to get out of there, quickly and preferably alive, and go home for a lie down. Instead I concentrated the mind and it was then I realised I wasn't there to get thinner. This bulk was what I'd become, not from overeating, greed or general excess, but this body represented the woman I really was. Big, filling a large proportion of the available space in the room, comfortable, even at times impressive. It has certainly been useful in my work as a radio interviewer. When guests come to the studio they're immensely relieved to find something other than a stick thin social X-ray sitting opposite them. Guests such as Monica Lewinsky open up to someone who has obvious sympathy with their size.

So I wear with great pride the signs of a lifetime of laughing enjoyment and the delivery of two fine (most of the time) young men. The bulk also helps belie my true age. Marlene Dietrich once said to a young actress, 'Darling, when you are young never smile – it causes wrinkles; when you are old smile all the time – it hides them.' It's a winning formula for those who are prepared to endure a diet of lettuce leaves and sparkling water, but I've always looked younger than my years, so to my mind the secret of an ageless, unwrinkled old age is to get fat – it fills the wrinkles out. Whoever saw an apple cheeked, plump granny who resembled a prune? Right!

So what were my objectives? I realised I had no real objection to my children's other chosen term of endearment – Miss Piggy. It was delivered with affection and trust, and even now as teenagers they occasionally like to cuddle up to the ample bosom – just as I remember as a child finding my grandmother's soft, yielding flesh a true haven (my mother is thin, damn it!). What I really wanted was to live long enough to nurture my own grandchildren, be able to run upstairs without booking a bed first in intensive care, and retain the energy and stamina of my middle years into the third age.

I can't, as I've explained, tell you my weight but I do know that I'm occasionally called a fat cow in the street (sod 'em!) and snooty assistants in clothes shops sneer when I suggest I might still get into a size 16 – so I guess I'm what would medically be classified as obese. In which case, 47% of the female population of this country is dangerously overweight, and in America the percentage practically goes off the scale.

Inevitable really when we consume meals with the calorific values required to work the fields all day long, and the only exercise we get is from the car park to the supermarket and back. But there is evidence that the constant droning of the medical profession about the health risks of obesity is wrong headed, guilt inducing nonsense – and that it is possible to be fat and fit.

Dave Alexander is my current role model. He's 19 stone and classified medically obese, yet he's a tri-athlete, superfit and competes at the highest level. Here's what he says about himself:

> I'm frequently described as the World's Fattest Athlete. When I turn up at the start line people stare at me strangely and presume I must be one of the spectators. But they soon realise their mistake when they see me set off with the rest of the pack. I have a fair amount of fat on my body, but I am very, very fit... We are conditioned to think fat equals unfit, but I am fitter than the average thin person. There are thin people who are very unhealthy and their bodies have a high fat content... Whereas I am in tune with my body. I have always been big. I weighed fifteen stone at the age of twelve and was regarded as too heavy to be in the football team. I took part in my first triathlon for a dare. The sense of achievement was so great I carried on. I train hard for every race. This means cycling fifty miles each morning before I go to work. I don't care what people call me as long as it spurs others to get off the couch and do something positive.

Quite. Dave is, of course, careful always to check his progress with his doctor, who now agrees that judging a person's state of health by body size is wrong. Dave's heart rate and arteries compare with those of a man half his age.

Don't let me kid you I've found it easy. There is no way I would dream of cycling 50 miles before work – it's still an effort to drag myself to the kitchen to make coffee. But the benefits came much quicker than I'd imagined. On that first day with Jason I managed only three minutes of desperate effort on the bike and convinced him I was having a coronary. Within weeks I could start as *The Archers* began (headphones are essential to stave off the ennui) and happily carry on until the cliff-hanger and theme tune – thirteen minutes at least. Then I'd skip to the rowing machine, then the cross trainer and even got the treadmill up to a fast walk for fifteen minutes. I haven't yet graduated to jogging, but quite rapidly I could manage half an hour of vigorous exercise, half an hour on the weights and then twenty minutes in the sauna. It takes a huge amount of self-discipline to get round there at the end of the day, but I've never once felt sorry that I made the effort.

Almost immediately people started to comment on the healthy aura I was emitting. 'My goodness you look well,' replaced the familiar 'Are you feeling okay?' I sleep better, feel less distended round the middle, drink more water and (a little) less alcohol, and while I don't think I'm any thinner, there has been a subtle redistribution. What was flab is still fleshy, but firmer.

It is boring and time-consuming, and there are weeks when I slide back to my old sloppy self or when the demands of the job, the children or the old man are just too great to fit in the time for myself. And there's the rub. The guys keep up the rugby, cricket or squash and never feel a second's guilt about taking the time for themselves yet that seems to be the hardest part for a woman. Guilt is our stock-in-trade – but it is better in the long run to feel racked by remorse at having neglected them and attended to yourself for a bit than to feel that awful nagging sense that it's getting too late and that coronary really is just around the corner. If you're fit and fat your family can expect to have lovely, voluptuous, cuddly you for that little bit longer.

And those shrimps in the changing rooms? You know, when you look closely, and I have, even the skinniest have cellulite – go see!

Seeing Bellies
dedicated to Judith Stein and Meridith Lawrence

Susan Stinson

Kitchen

>Come eat.
>I'll warm up rice
>with a fresh sauce.
>
>Remembering the moral weight
>of bread,
>I'll brush a slice across your breasts.
>Your nipples will press like cloves
>against your shirt.
>
>Leaving the tradition of a woman
>in the body of a cat,
>we become whales,
>all mouths,
>all surface,
>all grace.

(Belly Songs)

Most mornings, I wake up and run my hands over my belly. I linger over the texture of stretch marks, but the pervasive feeling is of live smoothness. I slip both hands underneath and hold it. Sometimes it is tender where it folds. It's always warm. My hands are drawn there. (*Belly Songs*)

I've been fat all my life. When I was 23 I moved from my home in Colorado to Boston. I drove across the country in a tiny car with two women I loved and two car sick cats.

Everything we owned was strapped to the roof of the car, which buckled in the parking lot of a roadside restaurant in the wide, flat state of Nebraska.

After my friends dropped me off in Boston, I was lonely. It was 1983. I saw a flyer in a lesbian bar for a fat women's group meeting at the women's centre. When I went to the first meeting, I walked into a room full of women who were using a language of fat liberation completely unfamiliar to me. They were all at least ten years older than I was. They were gorgeous and frightening. We sat in a circle. As we spoke there were undercurrents of passion of every kind.

I am in a swimming pool with seventeen fat women. We have our arms around each other's waists and are circling in the centre of the pool. We go faster and faster. Our bellies, breasts and arms press together. We lap against each other, screaming and laughing. The water rises around us. When we let go, we're washed against the sides. Sheets of water cross the floor. I'm drenched. My fat spills as always over my bones. (*Belly Songs*)

Some of the things I heard in that room changed my life for ever. I feel now as if I've breathed those voices into my own body, so that when I talk about fat liberation or read aloud from my fiction, when I walk down the street to the sound of someone yelling 'fatty', I am sustained and surrounded by the insights of other fat women.

For instance, the definition of fat oppression I use is modified from one I got from fat activist and writer, Judith Stein, who told me that she first heard a version of it from members of the Fat Underground, the San Francisco area group which sparked the fat liberation movement. It has also been shaped by a definition I read in *Overcoming Fear of Fat*, edited by Esther Rothblum and Laura Brown (Harrington Park Press, Binghamton, NY, 1989):

Fat oppression is hatred and discrimination against fat

people, based solely on body size. It is the equation of fat with laziness, lack of will power, deep psychological problems, with ugliness. This is a sexist ideology that works especially well to keep women in competition with each other and obsessed with what we eat and what we weigh. Fat oppression affects most of us whose lives have been touched by white Western culture, but the fatter we are, the more intense the discrimination.

Once I gave that definition to a reporter for a university newspaper. While I said 'hatred and discrimination against fat people', her article quoted the phrase as 'hatred and disgust against fat people'. I think this reporter was trying to listen with good will. That her mind inserted 'disgust' for 'discrimination' indicates how hard it is to talk about fat oppression in ways that cut through the intense cultural noise that fills our heads at the sound of the word 'fat'.

I hunched my shoulders and slipped both hands, palms up, under my hanging belly. I lifted my paunch, measuring the fat. Every time I took a shower, I checked how many fingers, or what fraction of a finger, was still visible as I peered down over my breasts and the gradual slope of my belly before it dropped off abruptly just above the first outcropping of pubic hair. Now that my belly overlapped my hands altogether, I tried to figure out how far it stuck out past the sighting point. It was the strangest moment of any ordinary day, standing there using both hands to hold a piece of me that wasn't supposed to exist, wishing it gone. (*Fat Girl Dances with Rocks*)

One of the places I learned to hate my fat body was at the doctor's office. When I was eight I took a bus to school. One morning I was waiting at the bus stop with the other kids, and a boy threw a dart at my belly. It hit and stuck. I pulled it out and looked down. There was a spot of blood on my shirt.

My sister walked me home. She cried, but I didn't. My

mother took me to the doctor. My belly was bleeding a little, and she was worried about tetanus. The doctor raised my shirt, and laughed. He said nothing could hurt me much through all that fat.

He was wrong. Many years of doctors equating my fat body with illness and death, of putting me on diet after diet throughout my childhood and adolescence despite the 95 per cent failure rate of this 'treatment' – of speaking to me with subtle and blatant disrespect, did hurt me. His words hurt. I never forgot them.

The woman leans back in her swivel chair. She's a feminist. She's at work. She takes a sip of diet soda . . .

I say: My fat does not detach. It has a motion like liquid. It moves in waves, it ripples. It is not a virtue, not a sin, it's a bodily element with its own purpose and beauty.

I'm an admirer of liquids. Water is a regular blessing, goes in pouring, keeps all human motions possible. Milk in the mouth is something with substance. It brings sleepiness, warms, fills.

But you're drinking hate in that can. (*Belly Songs*)

I was working as a secretary, but I knew I was a writer. I began to try to describe my own body, without judgement. This was not easy. In fact, it was obscenely difficult.

It was possible to begin to write about my body only because I had read the groundbreaking anthology, *Shadows on a Tightrope: Writings by Women on Fat Oppression* (Aunt Lute Books, San Francisco, 1983). I had read poetry by Audre Lorde, Adrienne Rich and Minnie Bruce Pratt. I thought Gertrude Stein's 'Lifting Belly' was a special erotic message, just for me.

In what I believe is a common condition in this culture – not limited to fat women – I was so disconnected from my physical self that I needed the guidance of great poets and to participate in fat liberation and grassroots feminism before I could describe or even truly experience the fact that my belly felt soft to touch.

When women ask me now how I came to love my body, I tell them that I looked at it very closely, and wrote down what I saw.

I sit naked on a chair with my legs slightly apart. I hold my bones very straight. My belly pours, hangs, moves, grows hair, shines in marks that fall like fingers curving up around its sides. I am loose, I hang. There are not enough names for the places where my fat gathers on me; there is belly, thigh, hip, chin, but no simple way to say soft-mound-between-breast-and-arm, or low-full-folds-that-are-sides. (*Belly Songs*)

I looked for chances to be with other fat women. There was a water aerobics class, organised by a fat activist. I loved changing out of my suit in the narrow aisles of the locker room with the rest of the class. Other fat women's bodies were a revelation. I was stunned by the specific and varied beauty of our physical selves.

I leaned down and touched the soft flesh folding over her shoulder blades. It moved like skin over water. Her flesh spilled out of the edges of her corset wherever it could. Bible verses were washing through my mind, along with a recipe for making soap, as I watched Martha sit up to unlace her corset. I couldn't tell where her breasts stopped and her thighs began. Everything swelled and folded. As she loosened her laces and her belly rose, I had to look away. (*Martha Moody*)

On a rainy day recently, I wrote until six in the evening. When I got up from my desk, I was tired, but filled with pleasure from the work. It had stopped raining. I decided to go for a walk.

It was a summer evening. The air was cool and light. I had passed four houses on the quiet street where I live, when a woman looked at me from her garage, then turned to say something to the man who was with her. He answered in a loud, jokey voice, speaking of me: 'If I ever start to look like that, *kill me!*'

I kept walking. The sun was muted. Tall grasses were rustling above red clover in a field. Leaves moved in the wind in a spacious, reckless way that always reminds me of the ways my body moves. I sat in the dirt under a bridge and watched the river. The man's voice saying 'kill me' floated away, but while I was writing the next day, it came back to haunt me.

If I start to look like that, he said, kill me. As if my life were a death. As if I should be killed. As if looking like me were both horrible and ridiculous. As if he could come close to assuming my appearance, even in his wildest dreams. As if the worth of his own life were so negligible, so fragile, that he would choose to die if his neighbours found him ugly.

It is painful to know that the sight of me represents terrible things to most people who see me in passing. Fat oppression hurts so many of us, but it is rarely acknowledged as a serious method of social control. The fear of being fat keeps women obsessed with what we eat and what we weigh. The pain of living in this culture as fat women – or as fat men, too, at larger sizes and in different ways – can be overwhelming.

She started swinging her arms and rolling her hips, the big swings of her belly moving the cream in a firm circle. Her hips stirred from the front and the back, and her arms caught the motion over her head and brought it back down to her hips again. She moved like sex, like magic, like the ocean she carried with her in her rippling back. The soft parts of her body that she couldn't agitate floated back and forth in rhythm as she worked. It was hypnotic and exhausting. Martha didn't learn so much motion in childhood, but grew into it with her breasts and the rolls of her sides ... She felt herself swelling, arms and belly spreading until she ... could move the whole sky. (*Martha Moody*, from a tall tale in which a fat woman beats a sky full of cream into butter.)

11

Even more constant in the lives of fat women than the realities of fat oppression are our soft, sensuous, fat bodies. I think of the pleasures of touching a fat body as a secret resource, an enormous source of comfort and power for fat women that we tap into when we let ourselves experience our own bodies directly, without all the cultural programming slamming down on our fingers and minds

> She made me tremble. She touched my body tenderly. She was soft and her waist fell and folded into mine. She gathered my belly in her hands, she rubbed her cheek on my small breasts, she pushed her loose breasts against my loose hips, and we were soft in mounds and extravagant in flesh. (*Martha Moody*)

The wonderful lesbian poet and thinker Judy Grahn, in the preface to her book, *Another Mother Tongue: Gay Words, Gay Worlds* (Beacon Press, Boston, 1984), writes about going to a library in Washington DC in 1961, when she was 21, to read about other gay men and lesbians like herself. She was told, by what she describes as 'indignant, terrified librarians unable to say aloud the word *homosexual*', that the books were kept locked away. Only doctors, psychiatrists and lawyers for the criminally insane could see them. The books were all written by 'experts'.

As obsessed as Western culture is with dieting and fear of fat, the same kind of silence makes most people too indignant and terrified to say the phrase 'a fat woman' aloud in polite company – let alone 'a fat lesbian'. So that, although we are incredibly visible to people who harass us on the street and discriminate against us in employment, access and health care, our lives and our bodies are rarely described except by so-called experts trying – unsuccessfully – to cure us out of existence, and people yelling hate on the street.

I believe in the power of art to help change this, to move people to grapple with complexity, subtlety and the evidence of the senses, and to evoke the emotional availability that is essential if we want to be able to work with each other.

My poetry and fiction include lesbian themes, but I believe that one of the gifts of art is that each life can illuminate every other life. I have been stimulated and stirred and recognised myself in art by women and men very different from me. I invite others to have such experiences with my specific fat lesbian sensibility.

Even writing and reading work about pain can be a gift, something that acknowledges a reality made more damaging because it is so often trivialised or denied. When a character in one of my books passes through pain, it keeps me honest and honours the resilience of fat women, all the work we do to find our various ways to joy. This is from the novel I'm working on now:

> Moonlight shone in through a parting in the curtains. I touched the burn. Covered with sweat, I could become it. I could be a blister. In my fat body, common as salt, people looked at me through blistered eyes.

In the years since I first discovered fat liberation and the beauty of my own body, I have written two novels, *Fat Girl Dances with Rocks* and *Martha Moody*. I'm deeply engaged with a third, *Fast Bus to Texas*. I've also written a collection of poetry, essays and short fiction, *Belly Songs: In Celebration of Fat Women*. The excerpts from these books throughout this piece are attempts to offer the heart of what I know about being a fat woman. There are rhythms in the movement of a fat woman's body that are as riveting and profound as any of the other basic rhythms of life.

> Two women dance. One wears a long scarf, silver and blue. Her black pants are loose and puff out across the form of her lower belly so that the waves in her body there, all of that loose rhythm, pass out through her fat and become

subdued and muted in the fabric. Her big hips send out currents that cross the paths of motion from her shoulders and her back. She wears a red shirt. It shines. The red goes darker deeper back in the folds of her fat, then pulls those hips up and they swing like power through the air, sending flutters down the pant legs, and her breasts fall like grace past the ends of her scarf.

The second woman wears no shoes. A new song starts. She is jumping, streaming colour. Her feet lift. The music sparks. Her calves are bare and pale under dark hair until the cloth starts halfway up them, strips of yellow orange, green pink, gold blue, sideways stripes that circle more and more leg as they stretch and quiver on up. Her ringed thighs shake, they bounce, they shake. She jumps. Her belly rises as she hits the floor, floats up full, tied in a white sash, big soft circle of cloth that could almost wish itself skin, but there are no wishes for cloth, there's just its properties: the colour, the weight and the width to give it a place wound tight enough for room for breath around so much wild fatness, making its own song in motion, making a song in largeness, the fat and the sash together up with ripples, down with passion, and the woman moving herself all over, even her chin is shaking, even her fingers dart and wander, even her clothes are with her. (*Belly Songs*)

NOTES

The poem 'Kitchen' on page 6 first appeared in *Bay Windows*, 1987.

The extracts on pages 6, 7, 9, 10 and 14 are from *Belly Songs: In Celebration of Fat Women*, Orogeny Press, Northampton, MA, 1993.

The extract on page 8 is from *Fat Girl Dances with Rocks*, Spinsters Ink, Duluth, MN, 1994.

The extracts on pages 10 and 12 are from *Martha Moody*, The Women's Press, London, London, 1996.

My Life as an Amazon

Stephanie Jones

I first became an Amazon around the age of 25. I had moved to London from Bath, and had spent my first few years here training to be a nurse and starving myself on a regular basis to maintain the hourglass figure I thought was my most attractive feature. My daily diet frequently consisted of a couple of apples, a banana, and a Mars bar or Twix. At the time I thought things could not be better, as I was young, thin, free, single and living in London for the first time.

Eventually, my body began to rebel. I realised slowly that the way I looked did not shelter me from the challenges and cruelties of life, and I could not maintain my starvation diet. I gradually increased in size from a 12 to a 16.

For a long time I beat myself up for having 'allowed' myself to put on so much weight, for 'letting myself go'. It also seemed that the worse I felt about my weight, the more I would attract people into my life who did their best to confirm my negative views. The downward spiral continued until, at size 18, I started to meet large women who were comfortable with their figures, who lived their lives fully and without allowing size to become an issue for them. I also realised that the only way I could revert to a size 12 was to restrict my intake to a few pieces of fruit per day. I was no longer willing to do this.

As I looked around me, I noticed just how many of my relatives were large – generally healthy and strong with it. My size was obviously part of my genetic make-up and something to be celebrated, not hidden. I have inherited my mother's amazing mezzo-soprano voice and wide vocal range, and I find that my size does make an immense difference to the power and volume of my voice. Simply put, I have found that when I'm bigger, my voice can achieve more.

Something that can be very hurtful is the reaction of slim women. I often have slim women look at me as if they are totally offended by my presence, and other large friends have had similar experiences. It is as if some women cannot bear to see a woman who looks good, or even better than they do, especially if the woman in question is larger. This must seem like the ultimate insult to someone who has bought into the myths about size and spent much of her life on a diet. I think this is because the confident, fashionably dressed and attractive large woman represents the supreme challenge to the size status quo. If large women can look as stunning as thin women without dieting, why then the need to diet?

We live in interesting times in the UK at the moment, because more clothing manufacturers than ever before have realised that big women do have lives, partners, careers, hobbies and interests, and want clothing that enables them to dress appropriately for all occasions. We also want fashionable clothes, trendy, elegant, classic, funky and sporty clothing in good fabrics, so that we can express all aspects of our personalities. In short, we want the range of choice that has always been available in sizes 8 to 14, and we want it now. I wonder what impact these improved clothing ranges might have on fat discrimination. It is easier to attack and belittle someone who is obviously lacking self-confidence, and if we are finally wearing what we like and feel comfortable in, that won't be us fat women.

I officially became an Amazon when I accepted my size and began to see it as an advantage, not a hindrance. By Amazon I mean a woman who is larger than the average, who is a warrior in that her size and its inherent strength serve to empower, rather than frighten and intimidate her. She believes in celebrating the many advantages of size. And she has an expectation that she will always be treated well. This, importantly, means challenging the negative expectations held by many big women who have accepted society's assumptions and stereotypes about size and unquestioningly put up with substandard treatment in all areas of their lives. Going through life with an expectation of being badly treated usually results in the fulfilment of that expectation. On a personal level, it has taken me a very long time really to understand this concept, but I'm getting there.

I continued to notice things that challenged most of the negative associations made around being fat. At Keep Fit, I and several other larger sisters always completed the class, while many of the thinner women retired halfway through. After walking several miles, I felt invigorated not exhausted. Most importantly, I began to question and challenge the Western standard of beauty that held all things thin, white and blonde to be beautiful. The evidence to support this challenge was all around me: I had been told that my extra weight made me less attractive but the enthusiastic reactions I received from men definitely put paid to any worries on that score. (Interestingly enough, I have found that my size is off-putting to some men, but usually those who are insecure and assume that size equates with being dominant and controlling. For other men, of course, this is a big turn-on, but I will say no more on this point!)

Size in the context of black culture is an interesting subject. Traditionally – certainly in the Caribbean, Africa and Asia – being fat has been seen in a positive light since it signifies conspicuous consumption and is therefore symbolically associated with good health and wealth. In fact, in many parts of the Caribbean, large women are still referred to as 'healthy' and seen as extremely sexually desirable. But this has been changing for a long while, and the Western obsession with size (and incidentally, with ethnicity and colour) is an extremely pervasive one.

Within African–Caribbean communities women, in particular, often feel free to tell someone else that they are fat – even if the person who comments is larger than the person their remarks are aimed at. A classic example of such a situation is one that I remember from my childhood. A woman called Mrs Ifield lived a short distance from my family in Bath. Now, just to give you an idea, my mum was a size 22, Mrs Ifield was a size 28. However, Mrs Ifield had no problem around commenting on my mum's size whenever we met on the street. The conversation usually went something like this…

Mrs Ifield: 'W'happen Jonesy, how yu do? But Lord, what a way yu put on weight, what a way yu get big and fat!'

My mum: 'Me all right Mrs Ifill. But how come yu always tell me 'bout me fat? Look pon yu! Yu much bigger than me!'

Mrs Ifield: 'But since me go pon diet, me lose two stone already!'

My mum: 'Well it nuh look like yu lose anything at all! Bwoy yu look fatter than ever! Is when yu really get tin yu can tell me about diet!'

My mum usually stormed off following this exchange, muttering under her breath about Mrs Ifield's cheek, and saying Mrs Ifield's head 'look like a mouse pon a one dollar bread' because her head was so small in comparison to her body!

I was reminded of my similarities to Mum in this respect a few years ago at the Black Beauty and Hair Show. I had recently won the Ms Big and Beautiful UK contest, so I knew I was hot! My Auntie Tiny (three guesses why she's called Tiny), who I hadn't seen for several years, came rushing up to me and started to tell me how fat I was (I was then a size 18/20) and how I needed to go on a diet immediately. She was so eager to start on me that she could not even spare the time to say hello beforehand. Unfortunately for her, I was more than ready to take her on, and informed her that as she didn't even remotely resemble Miss Slimming World, she had better take her own advice about dieting. She was really upset and told me that I was rude. I then said that as I had just won Ms

B&B, if she didn't think that I looked good at my size that was her problem. Auntie Tiny was mortified and embarrassed, as I had made these comments in front of some friends she was with. The fact that she had spared no thought for my feelings was immaterial to her. Needless to say, we have not spoken since, and she has told my whole family how rude I was to her.

More recently, young African-Caribbean women and men have also become increasingly preoccupied with the main-tenance of the size range that Western society has decreed is acceptable and of value. In recent years there has been an increase in the number of reggae songs that refer to large women in a derogatory way. For example, 'Oversize Mapee' and 'You too fat fat fat fat fat you wan go pon diet'. Although the songs are not taken that seriously by much of the black community, these seemingly humorous lyrics are then used by an ignorant few to harass and humiliate large women on a daily basis.

In some situations within African-Caribbean communities, such as at a dance or a club, it is interesting to observe the reactions of many men to large women. In the past, many black men would make their appreciation of a voluptuous figure very apparent, but these days they are less inclined to do so. Life in the West has strongly influenced their taste in women's shapes and although they might secretly admire a larger woman, peer pressure often prevents them from admitting this openly.

A fascinating development of recent years is the rise in what I call 'Fat Pride'. Within black communities this has been most noticeable within certain groups, for example the Ragga Girls or Dancehall Queens. As with many forms of music, a whole new fashion culture has grown up around Ragga, and Ragga Girls, regardless of their size, have been wearing outfits of a skimpy and very revealing nature, along with those liberally adorned with sequins and trimmings.

Amazing as it has been to see large women wearing such eye-catching outfits with confidence, somehow I doubt that this confidence is genuine. My doubts stem from the fact that a pretty aggressive attitude usually accompanies this supposed confidence, possibly in order to counter all the anticipated negative reactions to the wearer's appearance. Surprisingly, this woman does not tend to respond positively to honest compliments, almost as though she cannot believe the true intentions behind them. However understandable her reactions may seem, it is sadly not one born of confidence.

However, recognising how challenging it has been for me to feel able to step out in some of my 'non-conformist' outfits (i.e. 'not what a big woman should wear'), I long for the day when this process no longer provokes such anxiety or the reactions described above. And whilst I do have some reservations on the Ragga Girl's sense of style, I do applaud her self-belief and courage. I believe that she has been a pioneer, certainly in terms of changing what big women feel that they can wear. Interestingly enough, several less extreme versions of the Dancehall Queen look have filtered down into some of the more mainstream shops and I think are largely responsible for the more adventurous styles now being worn by big women. For example, the fashion for torn jeans and T-shirts started on the streets in black communities as 'raggamuffin' style and eventually became high fashion.

I think that the size acceptance movement in the UK often assumes that size is either not an issue for black women, or that it is less of an issue because large black women are seemingly more accepted by their communities. I think that it just *appears* to be less of an issue because one is more likely to see large black women who look at ease with their bodies and who are wearing clothes that large white women would probably hesitate to purchase, let alone wear out on the street. There is definitely a big difference in terms of what constitutes dressing up and appropriate dress in black society compared to that of whites. One has only to attend a wedding, a dance or other social function in a black community to see this, and many of the outfits I have seen worn at 'white' weddings are what I would choose to wear to work.

Certainly I would agree that attitudes towards fat in black communities are very different to those of white society, but I think that this has more to do with our differing attitudes to our bodies in general. A kind of celebration of the body, regardless of size, is much more apparent within black communities than white. Some might argue that this attitude has to do with the more 'earthy' (for earthy read primitive and exotic) nature of black people, but I really could not say whether this is true. For me, it has more to do with being in touch with your body and with a deep recognition of the incredible sensuality of fat, that delicious lusciousness that just isn't there with a thinner body.

Finally, always remember that we Amazons inhabit a parallel universe, a place where to actually look like a woman is seen as the worst thing possible, the ultimate disappointment. Strange though it may seem, our ancestors worshipped women who looked just like us, acknowledging our strength, fertility, beauty and unlimited potential for creation on every level. Who was right? I think I know.

Beyond Fat Liberation
Towards a Celebration of Size Diversity

Diana Pollard

I write this as I am today, objectively, unquestionably, a very fat woman. I am beginning with this statement because I want to make myself 'seen' before what I have to say is read. It may seem rather blunt, but I see no point in hiding behind words such as 'big', 'plump' or large. I am fat. Very fat. Indeed it is the first thing that people see when they meet me and very often the first thing they remark upon.

I am often abused, disliked, excluded and discriminated against for this reason. I am usually referred to as 'grossly overweight' or 'obese', and sometimes I am labelled 'morbidly obese', a term reserved for the very fat – people like me.

In knowing this one thing about me – that I am fat – people hold assumptions and judgements about every aspect of me. I have received unsolicited comments on my physical and intellectual abilities, my mental health, sexual responsiveness and even my honesty. I cannot think of another issue which raises such wide-ranging and unchallenged assumptions and prejudices.

As a professional counsellor working in the mental health field, most of the time I experience mental health professionals discussing fatness as pathology and equating fatness with compulsive eating and other disorders. It is rare that I come across a professional whose thinking has developed beyond having read Orbach's *Fat is a Feminist Issue*. Furthermore, even when the client has not presented her size as a concern, there is very often a hidden agenda held by the therapist, and weight loss may be viewed by the therapist as a desirable consequence of the client's therapy. I have personally heard weight loss cited as evidence of a good therapeutic alliance and as a measurement of a client's improved mental health! I have seen little evidence of issues concerning fat oppression being addressed, and when they are, they are viewed not as something to be challenged, but something to look forward to shedding along with the fat!

I can draw from my own experience to illustrate this lack of awareness. A gay counsellor regularly registered his exasperation that heterosexual professionals continue to make assumptions that gay clients are dissatisfied with their sexuality. I absolutely agree with his sentiment. It is absurd and oppressive to assume that gay people hate being gay and long to be heterosexual. However, this same counsellor had not worked through the assumptions he held about fat people. He had not questioned the validity of his view that all fat clients are unhappy and would want to become slim. His awareness of oppression did not extend to questioning the ethics of holding a weight loss agenda based on his own experience of happiness after losing three stone. For the most part I would say that counselling and therapy have a lot to offer and that many people find their personal power through the experience. But sadly, I do not believe this is the case for many fat people. It would appear that when it comes to weight, dissatisfaction is assumed and approved.

In the training of counsellors, a great deal of emphasis is placed on self-awareness of values and beliefs held, and accepting and valuing differences of race, sexuality, creed, class and levels of ability. However, with very few exceptions, counsellor trainers take the view that fatness is not part of human diversity like race and sexuality. It is usually lumped with alcoholism, drug addiction, sexual abuse and violence. It is therefore seen as 'reasonable' for the counsellor to hold an agenda for change. It is my belief that mental health professionals continue to collude with and contribute to discrimination against fat people in Britain, thus denying them access to unprejudiced mental health care.

To demonstrate this point, I will refer to the only book reference addressing fat, found on the suggested reading list of a university and British Association for Counselling accredited post-graduate course. In his chapter 'Fat Lady' from *Love's Executioner and Other Tales of Psychotherapy* (Penguin, London, 1989) Irvin Yalom tells the reader, 'I have always been repulsed by fat women. I find them disgusting; their absurd sideways waddle, their absence of body contour — breasts, laps, buttocks, shoulders, jawlines, cheekbones, *everything*, everything I like to see in a woman, obscured in an avalanche of flesh. And I hate their clothes — the shapeless, baggy dresses, or worse, the stiff elephantine blue jeans with the barrel thighs. How dare they impose that body on the rest of us?' (p88). And 'When I see a fat lady eat, I move down a couple of rungs on the ladder of human understanding. I want to tear the food away. To push her face into the ice-cream. "Stop stuffing yourself. Haven't you had enough for Chrissakes?" I'd like to wire her jaw shut' (pp88–9).

The views held by Yalom illustrate how deeply fat phobia is entrenched in Western society. In all his years of reflective practice Yalom fails to see the humanity of his fat client until she begins to lose weight. Yalom's ability to form a therapeutic alliance with his fat client is conditional, based on her compliance to lose weight.

In recent years some mental health professionals have challenged the treatment of fat clients.

In her book *Nothing to Lose: A Guide to Sane Living in a Larger Body* (HarperCollins, London, 1995) Cheri Erdman offers up a challenge to professionals working in the field. She asks, 'Are you willing to see this issue differently, to shift your focus from fat as a sign of pathology, to fat as a cultural phobia? Are you willing to look at your own fat-phobia and deal with it on a personal level?' (p158). In *Overcoming Fear of Fat* (Harrington Park Press, Birdhampton, NY, 1989) Laura Brown and Esther Rothblum (eds.) also challenge the fat equals bad equation. Writing from a feminist perspective they argue that the issue is *fat oppression* not fat, and that as professionals 'we must overcome within ourselves and our colleagues long and firmly held prejudices about the value of being thin' (p3).

In 'Fat Lady' Yalom is transparent in his view that he dislikes fatness but *hates* fat women. He reflects on how women should look in order to satisfy his aesthetic. His candid self-reflection may give voice to what many men expect of women. And in turn, offer insight into how women may come to judge their personal worth and that of other women on the thin equals good, fat equals bad equation. Professor Yalom is an acclaimed clinician and theorist whose work can be found on the reading list of many counselling and psychotherapy courses.

As someone who works from an anti-censorship perspective, I would not wish to see Yalom's 'Fat Lady' removed from reading lists. My concern is that work which challenges traditional beliefs about being fat and describes how fat oppression operates is missing from those reading lists. And I believe this is because reading lists reflect the biases of counsellor trainers.

In my own training I encountered many instances of trainer fat phobia. I was informed that trainers *empathised* with my need to hide my body. It was suggested that my choice to sit near the stairwell demonstrated a desire to hide and protect myself from view. I was disappointed but not surprised at this; fat oppression by liberals is often based on false empathy – 'understanding' that fat is unhealthy and that fat women are in hiding from their sexuality and personal power. Some time later this trainer disclosed that his entire family was fat and he himself was afraid of 'losing control' and becoming fat. I represented the thing he was most afraid of; his *despised self*. I agree with Brown and Rothblum that it is unethical for therapists who have not developed an awareness of fat oppression to work with clients on issues concerning food, eating, weight and body image. I believe it is essential that counsellor trainers have a clear awareness of fat oppression and address the issues in themselves and in training programmes for counsellors. Issues relating to weight and size should be re-examined by the profession in much the same way as heterosexual hegemony has been re-evaluated. As a matter of urgency, therapists need to look at the ways they equate fatness with eating disorders and their assumptions that fat, rather than fat discrimination, is their client's problem.

To create a picture of the world that I inhabit as a fat woman I have a wealth of personal experience to draw from. I have not always been fat, so I know how it is to live as a slim woman and as someone who has been various weights above the ideologically correct weight for women in Western society. It feels important for me to acknowledge that being fat has been the hardest thing for me to accept about myself (not surprising, when I consider that it has been the thing most frequently criticised by others). But I have come to accept myself and to stop blaming and punishing myself for being fat. I choose to see my fatness as part of the dynamic which exists between me and others and to make a challenge when I see someone relating to me in a fat-phobic way – to make the fat oppression in the relationship explicit.

We all live in a fat-phobic society and it is not just the slim who discriminate and oppress. Some of the most punitive attitudes I have experienced have been from those who were once fat themselves, and whose daily lives are a constant battle to control their weight, and from those who are fat but not as fat as me: it is not uncommon for people to oppress from a position of self-oppression. Within the relative safety of the Fat Women's Group a small fat woman told me that '*anyone* can find clothes to fit at Evans'. This has not always been my personal reality, or the experience of many fat women I know!

I have also encountered oppression relating to ageism and illness. I felt disempowered and saddened when articles from fat women describing their experiences of managing maturity onset diabetes and heart disease were censored out of the Fat

Women's Group newsletter because articles about illness were thought by some members to be 'negative' and 'depressing'. I believe that it is self-oppression that drives healthy fat women to marginalise other fat women's experience of illness and ageing. I question the validity of presenting an acceptable face of fatness. I see this desperate attempt to be perceived as always 'healthy, fit and fat' to be part of our oppression as fat people. Illness, ageing and death are all part of the human condition. Like everyone else, fat people do get ill and eventually we die. The question I feel compelled to ask is, 'How old does a fat person have to be before being allowed to die of old age?' Any celebration of our lives as fat people must be a celebration of our diversity; a denial of illness, ageing and death as part of this is to collude with our own oppression.

I have been involved in women's issues for a quarter of a century, and for more than a decade I have worked intensively on size related and body image issues, as a professional counsellor and as a campaigner and activist. In every area of my work with women of all shapes and sizes, two questions come up time and again: 'How can we celebrate ourselves when our lives contain so much daily pain?' and 'How can we begin to celebrate together when there is so much conflict between us?' I feel that these are very important questions and I have no definitive answer. However, over the years I have found ways of celebrating myself and also ways of celebrating with other fat people. For me, this has been a gradual process: from a celebration of self-acceptance to the joining with others in fat liberation, and now beyond fat liberation towards a celebration of size diversity, reaching a resting place – a place of peace.

There is an Irish saying, 'You have to know where you have been to know where you are going.' This applies to my journey to self-acceptance. I was in my early twenties when I came face to face with the enormity of my oppression as a fat woman. I had always seen myself as invincible, grappling with the challenges of my life, viewing it all as grist for the mill. I had grown strong to survive my oppression, but when I was told that someone who had never met me already hated me because I was fat, it pierced me. It is a long time ago but the memory is strong and still evokes sadness – the anger was dealt with long ago. I was left outside a new acquaintance's house while she went ahead to speak to her partner. Some time later my new friend revealed to me that she had needed to warn her partner that a fat woman was about to enter the house. I asked her would she have been so tolerant towards her partner's prejudice had it been racial. It was obvious that she had never thought about it in that way before and she was unhesitating in her response that she would not have colluded with racism. I have never spoken about this before publicly, and I am aware why: the partner was a woman, someone who was fully immersed in the women's movement and gay liberation. But somehow, despite all the consciousness raising, feminist analysis and revision of women's history, fat oppression had been overlooked. It was acceptable to hate fat women! It was for me a turning point on my size acceptance journey; a learning curve in the development of a politics of size. For my new friend it was the beginning of an awareness of how she, as a dieting slim woman, colluded with other women to perpetuate fat oppression. I was angry and I knew the reason for my anger. I needed fat liberation; I needed to own the word 'fat'. It was an important part of my journey and I have never looked back.

By disclosing some of my own experience, I hope to show that celebration for me is not about negating, avoiding or masking the painful issues in my own or other fat people's lives. I have come to believe that it is possible both to acknowledge the pain in our lives and to celebrate our diversity, talents and survival as fat people in a fat-hating society. I know from the work that I do and from my own experience that the issues are not the same for all of us, and even when the issues are the same we may experience them differently. What I write here applies to me alone with the exception of information that has been given to me by other fat people. I make no assumptions about how other people experience being fat. I am not comfortable with blanket statements, whether they are made by the diet industry, psychiatry or fat activists. Statements that begin 'Fat people are...', 'Fat people feel...', 'What fat people want...', 'As fat people...', suggest that fat people are a homogeneous group. As a fat woman there have been times when it has been important for me to feel part of something. However, I feel that this sense of identity is only strengthening if it is a movement which offers acceptance of all body shapes and sizes. What I experience is a sense of solidarity rather than sameness with other fat people. I use the word 'fat' because I am comfortable with 'fat'; it feels authentic. But I know many fat people do not feel comfortable with the word and choose to use other words to describe their body shape or weight. I feel the same sense of solidarity regardless of the word a fat person uses to describe herself – 'chubby', 'plump', 'big', 'large', 'heavy', 'rotund', 'chunky', 'plus-size' or 'overweight'. I have met fat people with remarkably strong self-esteem and size acceptance who describe themselves as 'overweight' and I have worked with clients who always use the word 'fat' to describe their bodies which they hate and abuse. In my view any celebration of size diversity requires a shift away from a narrowly defined ideology in which those who don't use politically correct language are excluded, derided and pitied. Our potential for celebration lies in the incredible diversity of the human form and the manifold ways of expressing this diversity.

The first Fat Women's Group was founded in London in 1987, and in 1989 it held the now legendary National Fat Women's Conference at the London Women's Centre (now known as The WHEEL). The conference was held over a day and included workshops on health, employment, sexuality, clothing and writing. Over the years I have spoken with many of those who organised the conference and those whose attendance marked their first experience of size acceptance.

The conference was a major achievement of the early size acceptance movement in Britain and for many women it was a formative and deeply empowering experience.

I experienced the conference as an opportunity to be with a large number of fat women from many different backgrounds. I found agreement and conflict, acceptance and judgement, similarity and difference, sorrow and celebration. For me the conference, like life, was full of paradoxes. It brought me new understanding of my own experience, and a step closer to the crystallisation of my own size politics. Some fat women argued that other fat women were not fat enough to be at the conference, and that they had somehow taken away places from other, more deserving fat women. I felt compelled to speak on this issue, arguing for the inclusion of all fat women. I was wary of being part of a movement which would hold a tape measure or weighing scales and stand in judgement of its members. I see this as body fascism, and I will not collude with the size police.

Not long after the conference the Fat Women's Group disbanded. Many of the most· active members were suffering from burn-out. The conference had been a huge endeavour, made harder by the media circus surrounding it. Many of the women who attended the conference went on to form local support groups and others continued to campaign as individuals. The first Fat Women's Group was a seedbed for many of the initiatives that have since taken place in Britain.

In 1992 a second wave Fat Women's Group was formed. Once again, its meeting place was The WHEEL. The new group consisted of women new to fat activism and some members of the first Fat Women's Group. Many of the women who had attended the 1989 conference, along with members of the original group, supported the new group and subscribed to Fat News (published 1993 to 1996).

In 1995, I received a gift of a book of black and white photographs, which was to play a very important part in my life. The photographer was Laurie Toby Edison, and the book,

Women En Large, Images of Fat Nudes, was edited by Debbie Notkin. I was entranced. To me, there is something powerful and empowering about these images and the knowledge that the fat women involved were in control of them. I felt an urge to do something of this kind in Britain, and I took my idea of The Positive Images of Fat Women Exhibition to the Fat Women's Group to see if anyone shared my creative vision for the project.

Tracey Jannaway was a founder-member of the second wave Fat Women's Group and shared my enthusiasm for the project. Other members of the group also offered help to get the exhibition up and running. Fuelled by our passion to bring the project to fruition, Tracey and I worked day and night for many months, and as each precious exhibit arrived I realised that I was holding history in my hands, and it felt like a sacred trust.

I have often been asked to define a positive image. I view this as highly subjective; therefore, for the purpose of the exhibition, we agreed on a simple definition: an image created by a fat woman artist or an image self-defined as positive by a fat woman. The emphasis was on choice and control, images which fat women found affirming, empowering and satisfying.

A short letter was sent out to organisations and individuals inviting them to take part. From this one letter developed a network of artists from many parts of the world. I was amazed not only by the level of co-operation and quality of work offered but also by the quantity. Until we made the request for exhibits, I had no idea how much talent and inspiration was out in the world, unseen images that could empower and make visible fat women's lives. The exhibition consisted of paintings in watercolour and acrylic, clay and wood sculpture, glasswork, photography, video, cartoon, poetry and prose and many artefacts from the personal collections of fat women. In the final days leading up to the opening, members of the Fat Women's Group, artists and supporters rallied round to get the exhibition open on time. Exhibiting artists included Sarah

Aleck, Lee Kennedy, Melanie Coles, Dari Walker, Laurie Toby Edison, Carlyle Raine, Karen Stimson, Ali Farelli, Tamar Altman and Megaera. Once the exhibition got into the media, new artists were contacting us the whole time. By the time the exhibition went to Manchester for International Women's Week in March 1997, Candice Farmer and Betty Woods had joined us.

No exhibition of images of fat people had ever been shown in Britain and it attracted considerable media attention. To my amazement, the day before the opening some of our exhibits appeared on the ITN Lunchtime News! At the exhibition we held an Awards Ceremony to honour some of the women who had made special contributions to fat women's lives. The award winners included Janice Bhend (editor of *YES!* magazine), Helen Jackson (campaigning barrister), Rita Jarvis (clothes designer), Grace Nichols (poet), Sue Surry (Big Aerobics), Mary Evans Young (Diet Breakers) along with other activists, artists and performers. Men and women came from all over Britain and other parts of the world. It was very much an international event with movement delegations from Germany, Sweden and France. Almost without exception people who came to the exhibition were enchanted by what they found.

The volume of media interest was phenomenal, with coverage in most mainstream newspapers, radio interviews and a number of television features – even the man in the local shop had heard about the exhibition. For the most part the media was remarkably respectful. It was as if they didn't know what to make of this extraordinary event. The memory that stays with me is of several women journalists who, I suspect, had been sent to the event with the intention of trashing it. I went round the exhibition with each of them before it opened and they were visibly moved by the experience. After the event, I was contacted by three of these journalists asking for my professional help on how they might develop a better relationship with their bodies. I was also contacted by several members of the medical profession – two hospitals and a number of therapists – all wanting to discuss how to work with fat patients and clients. One thing was clear – they had their doubts about the way they worked with fat people and they all disclosed some level of unresolved personal issues on size. They were all beginning to realise that they needed to find new ways of working with fat patients because their diet strategies were failing.

The level of interest in the exhibition and fat issues convinced Tracey Jannaway and me that it was time to initiate a national organisation for fat people. In 1996 we co-founded 'SIZE', the National Size Acceptance Network, a network of fat women and men in Britain. Three years of dialogue between networkers has resulted in a clearer understanding of our common goals, and areas where we have reached consensus are reflected in the SIZE Rights Charter for the Millennium.

Positive Health Care: The right to informed, specialised health care, focused on attaining disease prevention and optimum good health regardless of size. An end to weight loss treatments, drugs and surgery which cannot prove their long-term effectiveness and safety.

Employment Protection: The right to equal opportunity in employment. Potential employees should be selected on the strength of their qualifications and ability to do the job, not on a potential employer's discrimination, aesthetic bias, or insurance height-weight charts which are now known to be misleading.

Access to a Full Life: The right to adequate seating in all public places, including educational institutions, public transport and the workplace. The right to public provision of exercise and sports facilities and training, offered as a leisure activity, not as part of a weight loss regime.

An End to Size Discrimination in Britain: The right to see an end to size discrimination and to see size differences acknowledged as part of the rich diversity of a pluralistic society.

In 1998 SIZE entered a new phase when it launched *Freesize* magazine to celebrate its second birthday. *Freesize* is a radical departure from mainstream magazines, and once again I have been made aware of the huge wealth of creativity and talent of fat people which for the most part continues to be invisible in our society. The byword of *Freesize* is 'Freedom to be the person you are': its commitment is to provide a forum for dialogue and to celebrate and affirm diversity within the size acceptance movement in Britain and throughout the world. Contributions come from many of those who founded size acceptance in Britain and elsewhere, along with those who are at the beginning of their size acceptance journey. *Freesize* has found it hard to establish itself outside its own mailing list. Most of our support has come from women's and alternative bookshops, but they are few and far between. And, sadly, there are still 'radical' bookshops who refuse to stock *Freesize* because they see size acceptance and fat oppression as non-issues.

I decided a very long time ago that I was not going to put my life on hold until I lost weight. I have talked with many fat people on this subject and I have listened to many regrets. The champion swimmer at 14 who showed her medals at a workshop and who cried when she recalled the loss of the last 30 years without the pleasure and physicality of swimming. Teasing had left her feeling she must get slim before she could swim again, but aged 45 she had finally decided to give up the hope of dieting herself slim and had chosen instead to live her life in the body she had. It was a very powerful moment when she held up her new fuchsia swimsuit – an affirmation of her new full life. Then there was the man whose personal triumph was to feel safe enough to remove his jacket in the presence of other fat people after having experienced years of being mocked in the workplace.

I see every achievement a fat person makes over adversity as a cause for celebration. When I celebrate myself as a fat woman, I celebrate the very fact that I have survived and flourished despite all the things I was told I would never achieve because I am fat. 'You'll never be loved.' I am. 'You'll never have friends.' I do – and they are very special people. 'You'll never be a success.' So far I have succeeded at everything I have ever set my mind to. 'You'll never be taken seriously as a counsellor.' I am, so much so by some as to be considered quite a threat to the profession! 'You'll never convince anyone that it's normal to be fat.' I already have, including several members of the medical profession. 'You'll never be happy fat.' I am. I have learned that happiness is not a size – it's a state of mind. 'You'll never be desired.' Wrong again – but that would be telling!

I do not feel that I have been dealt a poor hand by being fat. I have my fair share of assets and advantages. I am creative, talented, intelligent, resourceful, passionate, loving, humorous (and of course modest with it!) among other things. I am certainly no shrinking violet. However, I believe that in a society where fatness is despised and thinness worshipped, many fat people do not reach their true potential because of the widespread belief that we have somehow already failed in life because we have 'failed' to control our body size.

When I hear fat clients speak of the negative messages they have internalised about what it is to be fat, I hear of the limited lives they feel doomed to lead as fat people. I believe that these messages can become a self-fulfilling prophecy and that *learned helplessness* is the result. When I am working with a fat client I am always working with fat oppression, theirs and mine.

One way and another I spend a lot of time addressing issues of fat oppression and working with the psychological wounds that fat people experience. I find the work both cathartic and challenging. Partly how I take care of and affirm myself is to bring positive images of fat people into my life. The images of fat that I usually see are stereotypes, with the exception of specialist magazines like *YES!* (1994–98). I rarely see fat women advertising fashion or anything else. When I see fat women in the media, it is usually an item about dieting or in some way they are being ridiculed. There are very few fat women in the media – Vanessa Feltz, Dawn French and Jo Brand – but for the most part I can go through my life seeing no positive reflection of myself as a fat woman. I believe that one of the most positive things I can do for size acceptance is to make myself and other fat people 'visible' in the world.

I have been fat for a long time now. I have known life as a small, medium and very fat woman. It is likely that I will be fat for the rest of my life. I am absolutely committed to living my life to the full. I have never been content to paddle at living. For me the satisfaction comes from being fully immersed in life 'Having said that, I feel that I need to add that as an intense, passionate person, life is not comfortable or easy for me; it has never been so. This is not just because I'm fat. I do not view fat oppression in isolation from other types of oppression. It is, however, an issue which I feel able to speak about not only from a political perspective but also from a deeply personal and passionate viewpoint. For me, fat oppression is first and foremost a humanitarian issue – one of many injustices that I see in the world around me and the one that people often seem to think in the scheme of things is rather unimportant. I am convinced that fat oppression is important, not just because it affects me, but because I believe it is a vital piece in the continuum of our personal freedom.

I see myself as a fortunate person. I have worked hard to carve out a life for myself from materials which I was encouraged to despise and reject. The work that I do for size acceptance is a way of celebrating my life and the lives of others in the richness of our diversity. It is my contribution to making the world a more size friendly place, which I believe is needed. What I do and how I am in the world is how I make sense of my life – it is what makes my life meaningful.

NOTE

All definitions of size are subjective. I see size and weight as a changing continuum. However, in this piece I have referred to 'small', 'medium', and 'very' fat people. I would define these thus:

Small: those above the ideologically correct size and weight

Medium: those definitely recognised as fat. They experience discrimination in all areas of life, but may have few access problems with seating, lavatories and other public facilities

Very fat: those for whom clothing may be a problem even in specialist shops and who have access problems and experience severe discrimination in education, health and employment. I would include here anyone whose physical movement is restricted.

Although all fat people experience discrimination and oppression in Western society, the less you are able to 'fit in' in a literal sense, the more you are likely to be marginalised and excluded from society.

Cinderella You Shall Go to the Ball
(in a size 28 sequinned evening gown that fits you like a glove)

Ali Jacques

Some time ago I was struck by the words of Susan Stinson as she performed from her novel, *Fat Girl Dances with Rocks*, at a reading in a London book shop. She swayed and lilted her words and took us on a journey over her rolls and folds as she caressed her body, inviting us to feel the soul seeping through her soft mass. The room was full of undulating sounds freed from this undulating woman in a whispering, Southern drawl. Then, for me, an awakening.

She described a shower scene – of soap, water and flesh, working up a lather on parts of her body 'which are not meant to exist'.

Simple, carved with a clarity that says it all – 'not meant to exist'.

Conjugate, Ms Jacques!

Parts of my body

Parts of your body

Parts of his or her bodies

Parts of OUR bodies

And how do we begin to celebrate something that is not supposed to be here? Something that in the eyes of Western culture has been pummelled into submission as the lumpy mass that dare not speak its name – FAT.

My personal journey, which took me to the top of the mountain where I shouted 'FAT' through an amplified megaphone, has been a sometimes painful experience. I have learned to love my despised flesh and, more importantly, how to deal with the rude and narrow-minded comments from other people who feel the need to impose their body fascism on those of us who do not conform to the Western ideal of beauty. Through that joy in my body I gained empowerment, understanding and freedom of choice. And fat is what I *choose*.

I was 16 years old when I wrote my first essay on being fat, imploring others to understand my anguish at not being able to find clothes I wanted to wear and how horrible it was being made to feel like an outcast. At school I read *Fat is a Feminist Issue* in the library when I should have been researching an art history essay on Egyptian artefacts. But when I should have been listening in on tutorials I was dreaming about the perfect life I was going to have when I reached my target weight. That was when the diet was going well. If it went badly (which meant eating an extra slice of 'tomorrow's bread') then I was hastily adding and subtracting calories. Maths should have been my finest subject!

I was drowning in a thin pool, floundering in the murky waters of body loathing and shame.

I have paid my dues in the realms of pain and paid highly. I – like so many women who have slaved to the rhythm of a thin alter ego – can talk wrist scars and Prozac till the cows come home. That is what is *expected* of us, to stay in our vicious circles, mulling over the years of hunger in bitter retrospect and comparing stretchmarks.

Well not today! As an adult fat woman, I now enjoy dressing my body to maximum effect, and I relish the curve of my belly and bum as they swell outwards in opposite directions, my shape expanding over the hips and giving me the figure that is natural to most women. So where was my turning point?

When I graduated, I made my degree film about the eating disorder I was suffering from and I knew deep down that I wanted to turn the camera explicitly on my own weight and size obsession. However, since the art college scene seemed to be into the much more cerebral and intellectual realms of art theory, I felt at first that this was an 'inferior' subject matter.

Who could possibly be interested in more burblings and moanings from a fat girl? So, I began to put out some feelers, talking in depth to friends and colleagues about their own diet histories and body image, and through this research I unexpectedly tapped into a wealth of women's experiences. Fat, thin or medium sized, nearly all of them were trapped in a personal, private torment.

The final proof I had that this was something greater than a group of women with nothing more to think about than what was printed on the label in their jeans, was when I put my proposed dissertation to my head tutor. He nodded sympathetically and explained that I would have to keep the argument academic and not focus on my personal experience, and I felt as if I would be prostituting a very deep and hidden part of my inner self to get through my degree. Then, as if to reassure me that he knew something about what I was going through, he said, 'Well, even my wife, who is a highly intelligent woman with a very responsible and well-paid job, always wants to lose nine pounds.'

Alarm bells ran in my head. *Even* his intelligent wife! His statement suggested that he believed weight affected only the stupid and working class, and of course, the most classic part was that he knew *exactly* how much she wanted to lose. This implied to me that she had probably told him countless times that she wanted to burn off that same nine pounds, and that she was obsessed with the detail of her body size to the extent of wanting to shed a specific quantity.

So, I began my dissertation, 'Eating Disorders in the Media: An Exploration', and set about delving into my own history of weight loss and comparing it to women around me. Dieting can be a lonely road, and so can bulimia, and I think in retrospect I really needed proof that I was not freaking out on my own.

Those I interviewed were bubbling over with the lava of release. Each had their own story which confirmed my belief that underlying body fears were sapping the creative zest and joie de vivre from so many talented and special friends who believed that their looks were essential to the core of their success. I needed no more convincing when a total stranger approached me in tears after my film was shown, saying 'that could have been me'.

Because I was hugely influenced by the world of films, fashion and fluff TV, it was impossible for me to ignore the increasing thinness of models, actresses, TV presenters and pop stars. Their highly stylised projection through the mass media heralded the dawn of the 'super-babe', and this prompted me to recreate some of the more instantly recognisable images, replacing the subject with a fat woman. I couldn't resist exchanging the tanned bones of a supermodel with my own white rolls of flesh, carefully imitating the exact expression.

It was of the utmost importance that the photo should be recreated using the same props, set, clothes, lighting, make-up and pose in order to eliminate the lame excuses people made when I tried to engage them in an objective discussion about pictures of fat women. They would say, 'Oh, the lighting's not the same,' or 'The dress isn't right,' and in my mind there was no point in giving critics an inch when they were definitely going to take a yard. I wanted to make sure they were discussing the issue – fat.

In January 1996, the cover photo of *Vogue* seemed to be causing a stir, and it was typical of the kind of picture I wanted to imitate. It depicted a naked Kate Moss tentatively perched on a sculptural red chair. The headline 'Nothing To Wear?' ran underneath her crouched and frozen pose, shoulders hunched to hide breasts beneath her cupped hands and her feet lengthened on tiptoe to elongate her legs, a supposedly desirable thing. My urge, as I twisted shoulders and cramped hips copying the position, was to sit comfortably, even if it meant 'distorting' the length of my legs, and I wanted to uncoil from this coy knot and fling my arms open wide so my voluptuous body was on display. I am about ten stone heavier than Kate Moss, and I bear her no ill will because she is a cog in a much bigger wheel and probably knows it. The fashion editor could have chosen one of several 'superwaifs', a new face, tomorrow's girl. What would a *Vogue* fashion editor make of my photos, I wondered? What would they really think of a fat girl daring to copy Kate, to think she could step into her shoes for a day?

Of course, I did not want to be a supermodel, and I disagree with the idolatry synonymous with their genus. I was merely trying to show what a real woman looks like in the flesh, sitting in an unnatural, silly position on an even sillier chair. The headline on my version of the picture was already in the bag. It ran, 'Nothing To Hide'.

Another image which was making waves featured Stella Tennant modelling Karl Lagerfeld's 'Eyepatch' bikini. Designed to celebrate 50 years of the troublesome two-piece, it was, as someone pointed out, 'three dots with a logo on it', consisting of a minuscule thong for the bottom half, and two milk-bottle top sized bits strung together for the 'bra'. With the black strings slung over protruding hip bones and the flat circles offering no use except to cover the nipples, I felt incensed that this image was supposed to celebrate womanliness, when in fact she resembled a teenage boy.

Once again I set out to duplicate the image, and I wore it with the best of intentions, to show a comparison. My message was, 'This is what your bikini looks like on an average woman.' It was never my intention to say, 'Thin is crap, fat is better'; I just wanted to see myself represented in the glossy mags I used to buy now and then instead of being made to feel so damn freakish and excluded all the time.

I created representations showing how I look in my underwear, because the well-toned torso is a highly used commodity in fashion and advertising and when a picture of a soft, womanly body is substituted, you can really begin to see the difference. I'm not condoning 'bare all' methods used to sell products, but if all races and sexuality and disability are to be represented, then body shape should be too. Let's see a size 18 woman emerging from the shower, applying deodorant and twirling in front of the mirror to make sure she can't see her sanitary towel. There are thousands of such images of size ten women, so why not show a relaxed woman who is confident with her fatter body? At present, fatter women are not at the starting line, and our absence is a slap in the face.

I also wanted to show real skin with all its blemishes, since we take for granted the million pound retouching process which nuzzles our qualms. I stepped out in front of the camera without a second thought of my wobbling cellulite and spotty bum. And although it was one small step for me, I truly hoped it would be a giant leap for womankind.

Gradually, more and more images began to appear in magazines which appeared to be challenging the notions surrounding female body shape, and I wanted to take my work further still. If a well-known actress could appear on the cover of a magazine showing her pregnant bump, what would it be like if I proudly held my belly out for the world to see? I have various theories on the attraction and repulsion of naked fat. It is easy to suggest that it is similar to the pregnant belly, but a pregnant bump is quite hard and unyielding, whereas a fat belly will move when a woman laughs, and every shape is as special and individual as the woman who owns it.

A woman who has just learned to love her body the way it is will want to share it with someone who wants to touch and caress her belly, massage and stroke her large thighs. Don't forget, these parts I refer to are not meant to exist but they do, and they are probably on you and part of you as I speak. Why should a belly only be celebrated if it is cast-iron flat or swollen in pregnancy?

My photos were never shown, but I plan to exhibit them someday. Although it was a liberating exercise for me, and a necessary part of my own 'body love', it occurred to me that I was merely recycling what were essentially stereotypical and misogynistic images of women, even though I was recreating them *fat*. At the end of the day, I was just copying someone else's ideas of what a woman is supposed to wear, how she should sit, smile, tilt her head to the left, pout...

My expressions became as flat as the paper they were printed on, and I realised thinness is *still* the decoy to distract us from all the other bullshit which is thrown at us, and how we are expected to find happiness in the length of a skirt, cellulite creams, the shape of a heel, the new black, 'Because I'm worth it.'

The photos were part of my evolution because I *needed* to see myself in those contexts to prove that, fat as I was, I could do it too. After all, the girls who were taking their clothes off for the glossies were landing presenting jobs in television, and that was where I wanted to go...

I vowed, like the Caped Crusader, to avenge the tyranny of women by the diet and fashion industries, and the best weapon I felt I had was TV, itself a fat-phobic perpetrator of female stereotypes adhering to the male ideal. When was the last (or even the first?) time you saw a fat woman reading the news? If it's not considered sexy then it should surely be considered serious. We cannot be stuck with funny and mumsy – the safe fat types which are supposed to represent all fat women – for evermore. At the least, I decided, things needed a little encouragement. And as a bubbly, camera-friendly young woman who loves to be seen, chatty and providing informative entertainment, I knew I was the woman for the job, despite the dent in my confidence caused by fat preconceptions.

Would producers (my prospective employers) take one look at me and assume I was slow and incompetent, and that viewer ratings would diminish if a fat girl presented the lottery? There are role models of course, but competition is tough and I know they work hard at developing their personalities to compensate for the extra weight.

Pigeonholing is an affliction all modern women have to bear, so how could I be sure my body shape might be the potential reason for rejection? They might think me too bubbly, the wrong colour, the wrong style, and I even knew of a red-headed news reader who was replaced by a blonde. Well, I wanted to try my hand in a world where I was almost certain that my fat *would* go against me, but it was a world I had always wanted to be part of, so I had to give it my best shot.

Unfortunately, producers usually have a fixed viewpoint of what a finished programme will be like before the filming even starts. And no matter what they might learn to the contrary during the shoot, they have their opinion and they're sticking to it! I have had several experiences of this, especially where a dubbed soundtrack is laid over the top of footage. Comments, both incorrect and aimed at having a dig, have been made suggesting that I would need half an hour's break after climbing a few flights of stairs, my actual weight has been notched up a couple of stone, and I've even had a soundtrack of a munching horse put over footage of me eating a cake! Even serious news features about fat-positive pioneers that I have taken part in have had 'Big Girls Don't Cry' dubbed over them in some way.

If the director has a fixed idea and I can't persuade them to change their mind, I will up the ante so it works in my favour and I feel as though I have more control, even though I know it may be edited out later. In fact, I get a rebellious kick out of being contrary and anarchic, and I'm much more likely to expose my belly or wear a revealing dress when I know that it's likely to cause a stir. I am always willing to be tongue in cheek about my size, but after a while I long for something really positive, to be included in well-budgeted, factual programmes which have a new and refreshing outlook on fat. Is that too much to ask?

I have taken part in a lot of features and debate shows, always as part of the content package. I hope one day to be fronting a show and that I can bring more broad-minded coverage to fat issues – both in content and presentation – because it never ceases to amaze me that those who are keen to produce original television can come out with a finished item which is identical to the last jaded piece of uninspiring reportage! I speak particularly of those programmes which purport to have serious and informative aims and therefore should know better – and what finer example can I give than the debate show?

After each appearance on these tacky free-for-all fests, I was left wishing I hadn't bothered. 'Guests' are deliberately chosen for victim credibility or for their ability to go for the jugular (the researchers give you a crash course in how to verbally attack fellow guests if you're new to the game). The presenters take a back seat and let it all explode in the hope that it will make great TV! So what was a sweet girl like me doing there?

Okay, I have to confess that I naively thought it could be a way into a TV career while simultaneously justifying why I had chosen to *be* fat after all my years of heartache. When vetted for suitability, I always made it perfectly clear that I was there to promote being fat and proud and that it had taken me a long upward struggle to achieve this peace of mind. Yet each time I went out there full of energy and enthusiasm on the subject, I came back feeling as though I had walked into an anti-fat trap and been ensnared unawares.

Don't get me wrong, I knew the format of the debate shows, and I'd even been shortlisted for a researcher's job myself a couple of years previously. I knew exactly what I was letting myself in for, but hadn't fully understood how very deeply my own fat experience went or how far we would be pushed into making that perfect moment of TV. So was it all my own fault, jumping in too soon and telling the world how great it was to be fat when I was really only just coming to terms with the idea myself? Well, when it happened, whatever stage I may have been at in my own mind, I felt totally exploited, humiliated and determined never to bare my soul to the media again.

In the build-up to one show I had let researchers know that I dressed to show my shape to its full advantage. They deliberately exploited this by persuading other guests to tell me how ridiculous I looked. This coincided with one guest, who had suffered terrible complications due to a stomach stapling operation, telling me that she'd give anything to be like me, but the audience couldn't hear this. I was moved to tears, and it looked as though it was the insults I was responding to. For the production team the result was a real coup, great for the ratings. I didn't feel angry about losing face, since I am a volatile, passionate woman who wears her heart on her sleeve most of the time anyway – but I was exasperated that the discussion had been reduced to a slanging match. It should have been a sensitive, compassionate argument and I was full of despair that such an opportunity for a real and meaningful debate about an issue that deeply affected the lives of all of us appearing on the programme had become a tit-for-tat row about clothes!

Eighteen months later, I had the chance to talk to a couple of publications about this experience and others like it. But since the subeditors had already decided on the angle of the article, I felt exploited all over again – powerless as a fat woman trying to tell *my* side of the story without someone controlling the scenario. Of course, in reality few women have the power to tell it like it is, and fighting for that right has become part of finding my voice.

The fat and sexy image was becoming a definite part of my trademark, and when deciding to attempt a similar show more recently I planned to wear something quite revealing, or at least to show my belly. This had the researchers running scared in the fear that I would wear something far too risqué for early morning TV (but I bet they wouldn't have objected to a woman parading a *flat* stomach at 9.30 a.m.). This time I took a back seat in the argument, deciding just to be that fat and happy woman while all around me were singing the praises of being thin and complaining about the difficulties of keeping the pounds at bay. I had realised that having to raise your voice over a studio audience is about as undignified as you can get. It paid off in at least one respect, as a member of the audience approached me after the show and said, 'You looked so happy there! Every time I looked at you, you were smiling and gracious!'

And so I am finding better ways of making myself seen and heard on TV. These include a sketch for BBC2's *Comedy Nation*, and my current project of writing a sitcom about three girls sharing a flat. In my work now, I concentrate on the interaction between characters of size, their relationships and experiences, which is a definite step on from plus-size photography. I'm not dismissing the power of appearance, but these days I keep that for me. I came to realise the hard way that very few women want to dress outrageously. The idea behind wearing clothes that are clingy or reveal more flesh is not to offend. On the contrary, my way of thinking is along the lines of 'come on in, the water's lovely' – especially after years of sitting on the edge myself, too scared to take the plunge. Most women have a very hard time coming to terms with their size and a positive body image, but women's attitudes *will* change when they want them to – and I am not forceful enough to impose my fashion sense on anyone!

I have learned not to let other people's comments grind me down, but to put my energy into striving to be who I want to be. I want to live my life as an active, outspoken and larger-than-fashion-allows woman of the world, and I have every right to take part in the feast of life. Cinderella, you shall go to the ball! So I'm going to treat myself to that dress, hold my head up high and *go*! Fancy coming with me?

Epiphany

Sally E Smith

When I look back at an early picture, I see an adorable, energetic little girl with hair the bright copper of a shiny new penny. I see her mischievous smile, her blue eyes, her look of expectation. I also see her chubby cheeks, her round tummy, and the folds of fat on her little legs, peeking out from below her dress.

I'm flooded with memories of my life as that fat little girl, and of growing up to be a fat teenager, a fat young woman, and a fat adult. Being fat has always been inextricably intertwined with my self-identity. And although I now use the 'F' word with pride, and I see 'fat' as an adjective, not an epithet, that wasn't always the case.

Growing up, I was given two distinct messages by my parents: 'I' – meaning my intelligence, my personality, my being – was wonderful; my body was a failure. My parents put me on my first diet when I was seven years old, on the recommendation of my paediatrician, who referred me to a dietician, the dreaded Mrs Hibbard. I remember her condescension, her rouged apple cheeks, her greying hair. But most of all I remember the 11″ x 17″ folded sheet she gave my mom which outlined how many servings of different food groups I was allowed each day, and more importantly, defined the categories and portion sizes. This sheet hung on the refrigerator, and I remember poring over it, trying to discover what I could eat and how much. To this day I can recite the vegetable portions that I was allowed: I could have one cup of french-cut green beans, but only one-half cup of peas or carrots. For fruit, I could have one small apple or one-half of a banana, and so on. Of course, I could always gorge myself on the 'free' foods, but how much mustard can one little girl consume? I discovered all sorts of tricks though, finding, for example, that eating the half-cup of peas frozen and one at a time made them last longer and was thus somehow more satisfying.

I did lose some weight; my recollection is that I went from 107 pounds to 70-some pounds. And I got a dose of the recognition which 'successful' dieters receive from those around them. The neighbours – who along with my parents had acted as the food police for the duration of my diet – were glowing with pride over my weight-loss achievement. My parents rewarded me by buying my First Communion dress, the first dress I owned that my mom hadn't sewn. And I felt whole and loved and powerful.

Of course, I soon regained the weight, which led to another round of dieting with a disapproving Mrs Hibbard. And another after that. By this time I was obsessed with food and tired of being hungry all the time. My parents would harangue me about what I was eating and would give me disapproving looks at the dinner table or simply refuse me when I asked for a second helping. I did try to outsmart them, though, by sneaking food when they weren't home or were out of sight. Furtively grabbing food compounded the shame I already felt from regaining the weight, and caused me to feel that not only was my body bad but 'I' was also bad.

There was also my constant fear of being found out. One experience I'll never forget involved the Ho-Hos my mother bought for my older sister. A Ho-Ho is a snack cake: chocolate sponge cake and icing roll, dipped in chocolate. I'd guess that Ho-Hos were three or four inches long, and they were individually wrapped in aluminium foil. When I thought it wouldn't be missed, I would take one from the box in the kitchen cupboard, and run out to the garage to eat it. My quandary, then, was what to do with the foil so I wouldn't be caught. We had an upright freezer in the garage, and I had the bright idea to throw the rolled up ball of foil behind the freezer. This worked fine for a few years, until I was ten years old and my parents sold our house – which meant that the freezer would be moved. I remember lying awake in bed, envisioning the wall of foil that would come tumbling down when my dad moved the freezer. It wasn't until a few days before we moved that I found out my parents had sold the freezer to the people who'd bought our house. I felt as though I had been given a stay of execution.

I laugh about the experience now, though I also find it ludicrous (and sad) that this young girl had to weave a (foil) wall of deception so she could eat snack cakes.

After Mrs Hibbard there was Weight Watchers, where I remember being berated by the lecturer for not losing weight while I was sick. When I admitted that I'd eaten soup (not bouillon, which was 'allowed'), she harangued me – an 11-year-old – in front of a room full of adult women. I vividly recall my face burning with shame.

Following Weight Watchers, during the summer I turned 12, my parents withdrew all my money from my savings account to send me to diet camp. Granted, Camp Olympia was no ordinary camp – it was six weeks of horseback riding, ice skating, archery, 'trimastics', and, well, hunger. And even though I got a 'scholarship', it was still too expensive for my working-class parents. But they were willing to go to any length to help their youngest child to fit in.

I had a great time at Camp Olympia, and I wanted desperately to fit in. I weighed 170 pounds, and I remember feeling sorry for (and somewhat disgusted at) Jackie, a 17-year-old who weighed 270 (or so said our camp counsellor, who made us promise we wouldn't tell anyone else this 'confidential' information), and who couldn't fit into our smart sky-blue tennis dresses with their matching panties. And I remember feeling jealous of the girl who was kept away from us for most of the time, the girl with whom the camp director sat all night in a showdown because she refused to eat her dinner and he refused to let her get up from the table until she did. Looking back, I now know the girl was anorexic, and my envy was misplaced. At the time, however, I wondered what it would be like for someone to *want* you to eat.

I never viewed my parents as ogres for wanting me to be thin; I had internalised that it was my fault, that I'd failed at dieting, and that my wanting to eat was a shameful desire. This was reinforced by the others: kids in the neighbourhood who would taunt me; teachers who would look askance when I bought a cupcake on 'Hot Dog Day'; and certainly by the doctors in my life.

When I was nine and went to the paediatrician, he told me to get off the examining table, take off my clothes, and bend down and touch my toes so 'I can see how fat you are'. I had never felt so humiliated, and I had never believed so deeply that I deserved that humiliation.

When I was 16, a different doctor told me that I was so fat that I'd never live to see my eighteenth birthday.

When I was 26, yet another doctor told me that if I didn't buy her liquid protein fast, I would drop dead of a heart attack.

I celebrated my fortieth birthday recently, and despite the predictions of these 'experts', I am alive and well. I do have an aversion to going to the doctor, however!

There were other diets; there were speeches by my parents (my father told me that his parents had kicked him out of the house because he was fat; my mother told me no boy would ever marry me, that 'boys only want fat girls for one thing'); and there was a consultation with a weight loss surgeon (but my medical insurance wouldn't cover the surgery, so – thank God – I never had it). But through these diets and trips to the doctor and hassles by my parents and taunts from other kids, I learned what I believed was an important lesson: it was so painful to be singled out as the fat girl that, if I didn't talk about my weight and if I convinced others not to talk about my weight, I could 'pass' as a thin person.

Objectively, this was patently ridiculous. Yet for the latter part of my teens and throughout my twenties it worked – and I could maintain a semblance of self-esteem by separating 'me' from my body.

I attended Loretto High School, a Catholic girls' school, where I was elected Junior Class President and Student Body President. These achievements wouldn't have been possible for a 280 pound girl at a public school attended by both boys and girls. Because we all wore uniforms, it didn't matter that I couldn't fit into the latest styles; because there were no boys around, it didn't matter that no boy wanted to date me. We were also taught by a group of wonderful nuns and lay teachers who instilled in us the knowledge that as young women we could do and achieve anything.

Thus, I was accepted at the University of California, Berkeley and received a partial scholarship to attend. Ultimately, I graduated from the University of California, Santa Cruz with a degree in psychology, though the two things I wanted to do most in life were to be a bartender and live in Alaska.

Throughout my college years, I expended a lot of energy pretending I wasn't fat. I lost 140 pounds at Santa Cruz, but I professed not to be on a diet; I was simply a 'vegetarian' who ate only salads and ice cream.

I was average size for about a year before I started to regain the weight, yet I still had enormous body shame. When I started to grow out of my Calvin Kleins, I was filled with self-hatred and remember crying hot, painful tears.

But my battles with my weight were my 'secret' life, since I still never gave anyone permission to talk about my weight, whether I was fat or average size, whether I was gaining or losing. Instead, I'd manipulate conversations around to other topics: my travels, and my hopes and dreams.

Throughout my twenties, my passions were my spiritual quest to 'find myself', partying, politics, the rugged outdoors, and the fight for justice and equality. The latter two stemmed from my father, who had died suddenly when I was 16 years old. He loved the mountains, and taught me to appreciate the beauty and magnificence of the Sierra Nevadas. Inadvertently, he also taught me about justice and equality when he forbade me to play with a school friend because she was black. Never mind that her dad was a rich doctor and my dad was a working-class construction foreman. I was furious, and through my 12-year-old eyes I saw very clearly the immorality of racism and injustice.

In the years following college graduation, I had an eclectic mix of jobs. First, I was a computer operator for a company I had worked for during summer vacations. They didn't want to lose me and offered to send me to programmer's school, but working with computers didn't give me any sense of spiritual or emotional well-being. So from there I went to work for the California legislative office of the American Civil Liberties Union, an organisation which fights to protect and uphold the US Constitution and Bill of Rights. I was in the thick of the political arena, which I loved, and worked for issues I believed in: the rights of the accused, free speech, privacy and reproductive rights. I felt as though I was contributing to society (a lesson I'd learned from my mom, who though a political conservative was a 'professional volunteer' for most of my childhood), and thus could sleep well at night. I also spent many evenings at the Torch Club, a somewhat seedy bar where everyone from politicos to street people hung out.

The Torch Club also gave me an opportunity to fulfil my dubious wish to become a bartender with some real on-the-job training. It was a place where a 220-pound young woman could be a cocktail waitress, thus reinforcing my perception that I could 'pass' as a thin person.

But in November 1983, I went to Alaska to visit a girlfriend who had moved to Anchorage and I heard the siren song of the wilderness. I happened to meet a man who was visiting the city from his job rebuilding a fishing lodge out in the mountains. He said he wanted a partner in his endeavour and that I filled the part. I came back to California, quit my job at the ACLU, sold everything I owned, and moved to Alaska in January. When I stepped off the plane it was -22° and I knew – to paraphrase Dorothy from *The Wizard of Oz* – that I wasn't in Kansas any more. Flying in the bush plane and landing on skis on a frozen lake was quite an experience, as was living without running water or electricity in the middle of an Alaskan winter. Melting snow for bathwater, avoiding angry moose, and learning other survival skills was quite an adventure and gave me a degree of self-confidence that few other experiences could. The view of Mount Denali (McKinley) from the front window on a clear day, the crisp coldness of the air, and the sheer isolation gave me a sense of peace and tranquillity that would be difficult to duplicate.

Eventually I moved back to California, where I worked again as a bartender until I networked with the lobbyist for the building trades, who offered me a job as a construction labourer. He said the labourers' union was trying to get more women to join, which for me triggered the possibility of fighting my feminist battles on the front line, and he also said the starting pay was $16 an hour, which clinched the deal.

My three years as a labourer were filled with much hard work and many lessons. I'd always considered myself a feminist, and identified with women's oppression, but because I'd always tried to 'pass' as a thin person I'd never identified with the oppression of fat people. That is, not until one hellaciously hot day on a construction site. There was one other woman besides myself on the crew; she looked as though she could have stepped out of *Playboy* magazine. Perfect nails, perfect long dark hair, teeth that were whiter-than-white, skin-tight jeans and brand-new boots. It was her first day on the job, and as she was flagging traffic in the cool, crisp morning, she almost caused an accident. I noticed the foreman taking more than a passing interest in his new crew member. The day got warmer, and before long my 'sister' in the crew was riding around the foreman's air-conditioned truck, while

I wrestled with a jackhammer in the sweltering heat.

At that moment, it struck me like a bolt of lightning that this wasn't about women's oppression, it was about fat oppression; that the foreman never gave me a second glance because I weighed 250 pounds, but let her slack off because she was thin, buxom and good-looking. This was my epiphany as a fat person. I was used to fighting the injustice and oppression that other groups face, but I'd so internalised the messages of self-hatred and shame that are pounded into fat people that I never stopped to consider that we are also disenfranchised.

This pivotal experience didn't mean that I hopped 'out of the closet' overnight, but rather that I had begun a process that would become impossible to reverse.

It wasn't long after that I read an account by advice columnist 'Dear Abby' about NAAFA, an organisation that advocated for the rights of fat people. I remembered hearing about the organisation when I was young, on a segment of the TV show *60 Minutes*. Back then, I was morbidly fascinated by such an organisation, but mystified as to how those people could be fat and proud. But at this point, I was ready to find out more so I wrote and asked for information.

I joined NAAFA shortly thereafter, but I was still 'in the closet'. I was still ashamed of myself, and somewhat ashamed of belonging to an organisation for fat people. I'd keep my newsletters tucked away so my boyfriend (and soon-to-be husband) wouldn't see them. I would read them over and over again, questioning if everything I'd been taught about my body and about fatness could possibly be wrong.

Over the next year or so, I pretty much stopped dieting (although my last diet, the Rotation Diet, would result in a 25-pound weight loss). I also got married, designed and supervised the building of our home, decided I'd worked enough construction for one lifetime, and went to work for the Lobby for Individual Freedom and Equality – an organisation that lobbied for responsible AIDS legislation.

In mid-1997 there was an article in the NAAFA newsletter that said the organisation, based in New York, needed an executive director in order to reach its level of growth, but that NAAFA didn't have the money to hire one. I read that article and decided on the spot that I was going to be NAAFA's executive director. I wrote a lengthy letter to the board of directors, which was basically a thinly-veiled résumé, outlining why an executive director did not need to be based in New York, and how they should try to find someone who had the wherewithal to work initially without a salary.

My letter led to a series of discussions with various members of NAAFA's leadership, an ongoing dialogue in which I became more familiar with the organisation and its players, and they came to know me better. That fall, I wrote a proposal to the board that they hire me as executive director, offering to work without pay until I could raise enough money for my salary. This culminated in my flying to New York for NAAFA's board meeting, which was held in conjunction with the organisation's Holiday Happening – a fundraising event with workshops, speakers and dances, which was held over the New Year weekend.

I'd never been around many fat people before. Indeed, I had done my best to avoid ever being seen with another fat person. With all my efforts to 'pass' as a thin person, the last thing I wanted was to be associated with anyone else who was fat. So when I walked into the hotel ballroom for the dance, and witnessed 200 people all sizes of large who were dressed to kill, the sight took my breath away. I had my second epiphany, overwhelmed by the feeling that these were my people, that I'd come 'home' and I never had to hide again.

I walked into the board meeting on 1 January 1998, and after a few perfunctory questions was hired as the organisation's first executive director. That moment changed my life irrevocably.

Since that day, I have had experiences I could never have dreamed of. I've done over 2000 media interviews, including two appearances on *Larry King Live*. I've met with Mario Cuomo, the then-Governor of New York. I've organised a demonstration at the White House, planned conferences for 500 attendees, talked with the National Institutes of Health about obesity-related public-health policy, and spoken at conferences sponsored by both the Harvard Medical School and Stanford Medical Schools. I've travelled to at least half of the USA's 50 states, as well as to Belgium, to spread the message of size acceptance. I've written over 50 articles for publication and have talked to everyone from teachers to psychiatrists about the myths and stereotypes about fat people.

And as for my personal journey, I've lived through divorce, the death of my mother, the birth of my beautiful son, and the many highs and lows that occur on the rollercoaster of life.

I'm also still on the path of learning to love and value myself, regardless of my size. Certainly, the self-hatred about my fatness has gone out the window, and my 'fat and ugly' days only occur once a year or so instead of every day. But I adhere to Cheri Erdman's theory that the process of self-acceptance is a spiral; that we come around to work through the same issues again and again, on ever-deepening levels.

For example, I'd assumed that I'd worked through my mind/body dichotomy, where 'I' was good and my body wasn't. I loved my round, abundant body and enjoyed that my partner adored it and found me sexy and provocative. Yet three years ago when I was pregnant, I discovered that I had no confidence that my body could produce a healthy baby; rather, I had a deep-seated feeling that my body was rotten inside. I was shocked to uncover this conviction, and had a difficult time being able to trust the ability of my body to nurture this new life. Likewise, though I loved my body size and shape, when my body began to change with pregnancy, it took me a while to come to terms with and love my new shape, as well as with my post-pregnancy body.

Another continuing struggle is facing the challenge of believing 'I'm worth it', whether that means receiving unbiased medical care, demanding seating that fits me, confronting prejudiced attitudes of people I meet, or taking the steps to treat myself well. I've so internalised the message that I'm a second-class citizen – that somehow I'm 'less than' the thin people in this world – that demanding my rightful place in society is sometimes an effort.

Yet when I look back, I see how far I've come from that ashamed little girl I once was. And when I look around, and witness how both average size and fat women engage in body hatred and put their lives on hold waiting to be thin or thinner, I celebrate my continuing journey and wish that I could gather all of my fat sisters and brothers in an embrace – to let them know that this exciting, scary journey is worth the risk.

Fat Fantastic

Lee Kennedy

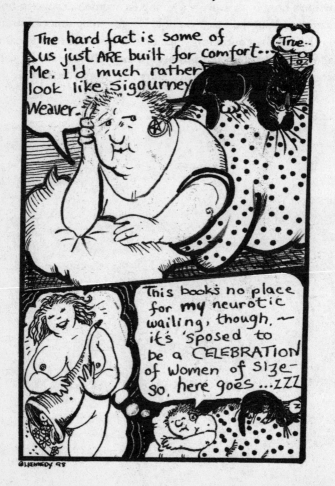

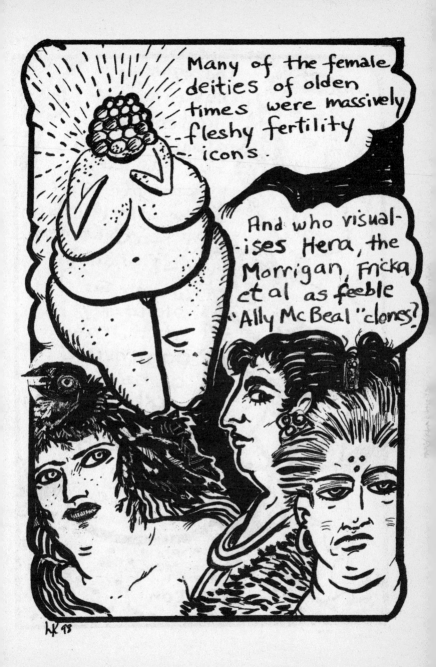

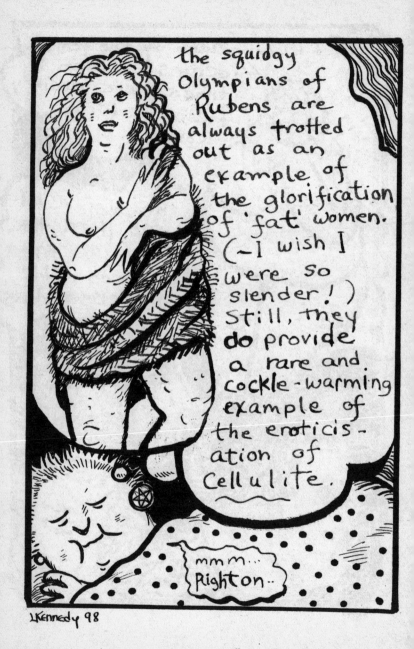

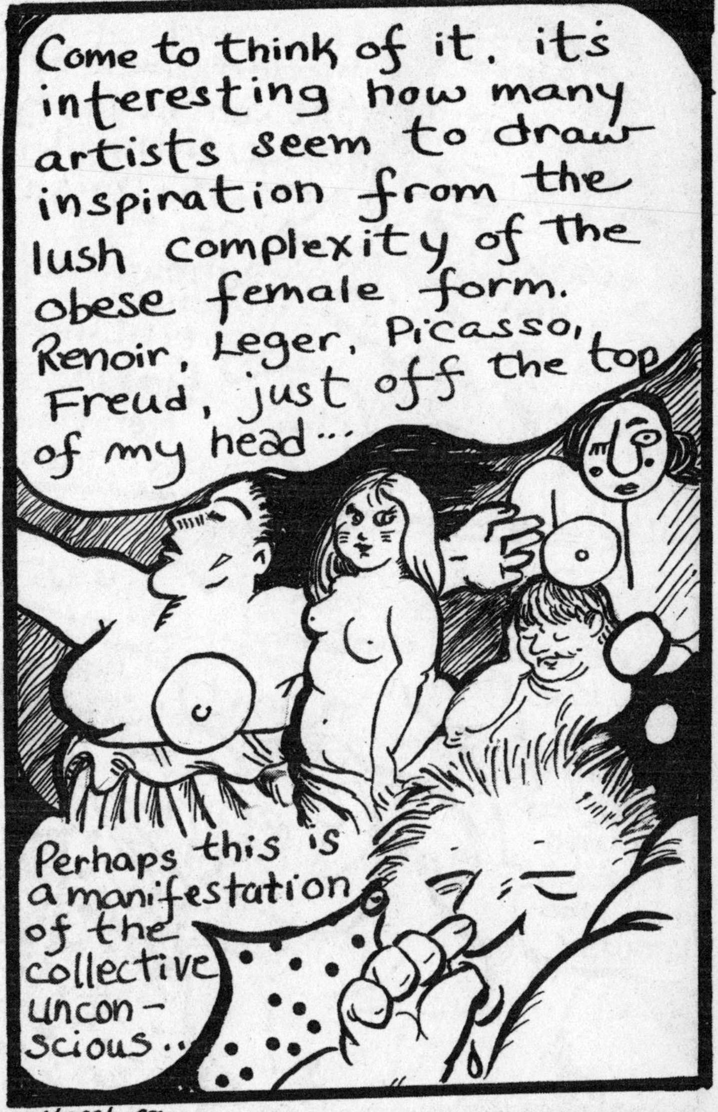
Come to think of it, it's interesting how many artists seem to draw the inspiration from the lush complexity of the obese female form. Renoir, Leger, Picasso, Freud, just off the top of my head...
Perhaps this is a manifestation of the collective uncon-scious..
LEE KENNEDY 98

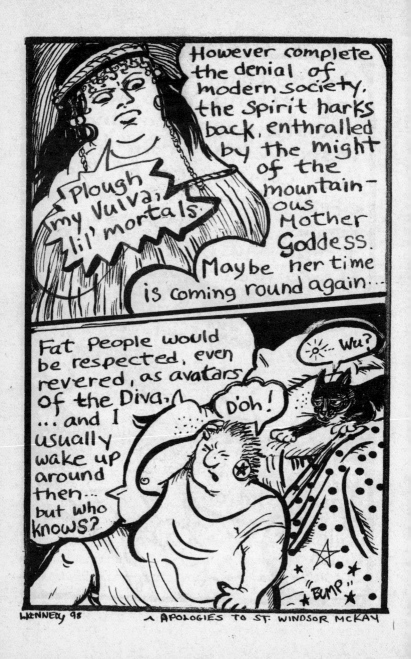

The Sugar Plum Fairy's Progress

Kathryn Szrodecki

'Kathryn, are you sure you passed?' she asked incredulously. I paused in the telling of my good news and stared at her; she rephrased her question. 'Did they really pass you?' I stared at her again, looking into her face for clues. Had she not heard me, or was I gabbling out my wonderful news in such a way that I simply hadn't made sense?

'This was the YMCA – the examiners, I mean?'

'Yes,' I replied.

'It was,' she nodded, 'it was the YMCA?'

'Yes.'

'And they passed you?'

'*Yes.*' The smile started to slip from my face as the reality of her questioning hit me. Here I was, 200lbs and telling my friend the aerobics instructor of 110lbs and–proud–of–it that I had just achieved the same qualification as her.

A wave of sympathy for her rolled over me; her world had just slipped on its axis. The governing body of her profession had made a leap in consciousness she was not ready for. Aerobics instructors are supposed to be thin, she was sure of that, and now my news had rocked the foundations of her life. A snap of anger was locked between her eyes, furrowing her brow. Daily she fought the good fight against body fat, she dieted, and at the looming shadow of any extra poundage she doubled her exercise routine. Dammit, she had worked bloody hard to achieve and maintain the size eight to ten body necessary for an instructor, and here was Kathryn, big fat

Kathryn, telling her that the YMCA regarded them as equal. This was not fair, there must be some mistake.

She took a step back from me, the shock on her face naked and pained, as she realised that I was telling the truth. Something had changed for ever, we hardly spoke again. Then she moved to South Africa.

My YMCA examiners had told me that I was the first larger sized instructor they had passed. I think they surprised themselves. The fitness industry has been one of the leading perpetrators of the body myth that a size ten is available to everyone: if you harness your self-discipline and focus your determination you too can have the current ideal body. This is a lie.

The true point has been missed. Exercise is about getting active enough to ensure that your body is working and serving you in your life, giving you its best performance on demand. And the payoffs of greater activity are vast: better circulation, stronger heart, greater lung capacity, stronger muscles, stronger bones, less risk of osteoporosis – as you can tell, I could go on! The truth is, regular exercise, whatever your hip size, is possibly the most crucial and important single thing you can do today to radically improve your overall health.

I am sitting down to write this having travelled 200 miles home from a conference on Diet and Nutrition, where I have spent the day listening to a string of leading scientists illustrate, with slides, how dangerous it is to be obese. One said that probably the only way to stem the rising epidemic of obesity was to pick up a kalashnikov and massacre as many fat people as possible. For me that was as close an admission to failure on the part of the scientists (most of whom are bought and paid for by the drug companies who produce diet drugs and associated products) as we are going to hear. It occurred to me that I was watching Custer's last stand today; the Indians are massing on the hills, listen to the smoke signals.

Obesity is not a disease; it's an insult. Those of us with larger hips are not failures and medical risks; we are in fact nature's success stories. For most of the population of the West, this is the first era where we have had something approaching full nutrition and the majority are financially able to eat a lot better than their grandparents. This has its drawbacks, for with greater access to food has come poorer quality. It is still possible to be malnourished on our over-processed food, and we also burn less fuel in our daily activities. For centuries food was seasonal, and a poor crop meant a hungry winter. Therefore the section of the population most likely to survive a hard cold winter with short rations was those who metabolised their food the most efficiently, who easily converted and stored food for future use. That's us, the fat ones! Centuries of uncertain food availability amongst all but the smallest percentage of our society led people to view the larger body with desire and admiration. Don't forget this in the insane confusion of body falsities which surround us; if we ever face the destiny of the dinosaurs we, the fat ones, will probably be the last to become extinct.

And on the subject of insanity, have the doctors ever peered at you, casting their eyes over your body, fully white-coated and licensed-to-judge, drawn back and said: 'Maybe you need a bit more self-control, dear, a bit of self-discipline, eh?' then continued, circling and assessing their victim with pursed lips.

'You are shortening your life by several years, you know, carrying all this fat' (as if we have made a steady increase in hip size our life's ambition), and encouraged by your discomfort, sensing blood, they crouch, waggling their bottoms (cat-wise), poised to pounce.

'Do you have children?' they ask with tilted head. 'How will they feel when you're dead?' Triumphantly they give a thin smile.

The joke is you only went to see them for an ingrown toenail. No wonder we larger women consistently have cervical smears and other investigations less frequently than our thinner sisters.

Trust me, they don't know what they're talking about; don't

let the white coat fool you. This easy equation of calories in, calories out, holds no water. We are far more complicated than that; we are not car engines as they would have you believe. Our energy systems are complex and overlapping and reliant on all kinds of factors, and it's the same with generalisations about heart disease; if having big hips equals heart disease, then why do so many thin people have heart attacks? Report after report is being published by scientists who care enough to do a study, often of thousands of people over decades, all saying the same thing: those of us who are active with a stable body weight – whatever size we are – live the longest and have the least risk of disease. When will the medical profession read their own research? Perhaps when a stomach stapling surgeon passes through the eye of a needle.

Ninety per cent of body size and shape is genetically determined. If you take a naturally large person, feed them denatured, over-processed food, add a more sedentary lifestyle, watch them get larger, then 'cure' them by alternately starving them and refeeding them regularly over a period of years, then hey presto! you have a prescription for disaster, a body hopelessly out of tune with itself, possibly with a damaged immune system, suffering from decades of stress related illness. Yes, sometimes we are more unhealthy than our thinner counterparts, but is it the fat which is to blame, or the 'cure' for the fat?

Dieting has damaged our health; the delicate balance of our bodies cannot withstand repeated or constant semi-starvation. Often the larger person with health challenges is simply dealing with starvation induced disease. The mythical 'tremendous benefits to health achieved with 10% weight loss' touted by the diet drug barons is nothing compared to the long-term damage several months of dieting can produce. The greatest contribution you can make to your health is to eat well and increase your physical activity.

As a child I wanted to be a ballerina. I went to the *Nutcracker Suite* as a treat after a nasty dose of German Measles. Ahh! this was it, that was me, there in the mauve tutu – sugar plum fairy me. Unfortunately my brother turned that neatly into fairy elephant as my obsession grew and I could be found pirouetting and pas de chat-ing on the lino in the living room. I found lino gave my movements that gliding grace necessary for the sugar plum fairy. I didn't have a tutu or point shoes, but I had lino – watch me glide! Eventually, fearing for their flooring, my parents gave me lessons. At age four, I went to classes. I loved it. In my pink tights and leotard I was a star, the queen of ballerinas. I stayed for six years, didn't miss a class.

I never understood why they told me I was too big to be a dancer. It didn't make sense – I could do all the exercises, I was good. But they said no, there was no point in my taking the exams, I was too large, and they shook their heads and looked with a mixture of fondness and repulsion at me.

'This is not for you, dear, dancers have to be delicate, light things, so the men can lift them, you see. They couldn't lift you now, could they? You'd squash them.' They added a smile and a slight lean forward, hands clasped and resting near the knees, to soften the blow of harsh reality in my 11-year-old world.

What saved my sanity at this point in my life was the complete lack of truth or logic in their argument: that men's lifting ability had to define who shall dance and who shall sit and watch did not hold water for me. As I saw it, only one dancer got lifted and there were plenty of others on the stage dancing away unlifted. What, so they had to be thin just in case the man dancer had a fit and decided to lift them all, one at a time? And what about my ability to dance, didn't that count? That I was strong, flexible and poised? Not enough, I guess – it was my hip size that counted. What nonsense. I simply did not believe them; the ratio of lifted to unlifted dancers was 1 to 100. Why could I not be one of the one hundred, I asked and they placed the final straw. 'They don't make tutus big enough for you, dear.' A tight smile: 'Sorry', and I gave up ballet.

Physical activity should not be the privilege of the thin. As larger people we have been denied the joy of movement for too long. Fear of humiliation, shame and exclusion have kept us hidden. For me exercise is a way to 'come out' and declare myself as fat and fully participating in life. I try to deny myself nothing and run eagerly towards each new experience; I feel the joy of showing up again in my life. To be fully present, alive and in love with myself again, and to try and retain this with grace, even in the face of most of the medical profession and the entire fitness industry – that, for me, is self-discipline; *that* is self-control.

Still on the subject of insanity, I thought that perhaps we were gaining some ground with the holistic, self-development, wise-woman, new-age movement. I thought that hip size would slip back into proportion with this new focus on mind, body and spirit, that maybe we could relax a bit with all this healing that's going on, with our eyes set firmly on the energy, not the form, for a change. I thought if I just forgave my parents, got regular crystal therapy, meditated a lot, and eschewed all things chemical, I'd be in there, a fully paid up member, a bona fide accepted woman/goddess. Well, not a bit of it. You see, unfortunately fat is just as unpopular amongst new age therapists as it always has been amongst old age therapists. It appears that you can't be enlightened and fat.

As 'those on the path' will happily tell you, your fat is a symptom of deeper problems, an indication of your unhealed childhood trauma/repressed sexuality/anger at your mother. Of course thin people don't have these problems. And if you look enquiringly at them and let them bang on a bit, they'll go further, waxing lyrical about us having to protect ourselves with a body armour of fat to keep people away, a bit like visual halitosis. Even Marianne Williamson, who was one of my personal favourites for a while given that I am a Course in Miracles student, states '... and all fat women are so because they don't believe they deserve to be thinner.' What? She would never write 'All short people are so because they don't believe they deserve to be taller', or 'All Chinese are dark-haired because they don't believe they deserve to be blond', or 'All men are men because they don't believe they deserve to be women.'

Overeaters Anonymous sum it up: 'Thinness will not make you well, but wellness will make you thin.' As with the previous theories, this enchanting slogan presupposes that being thin is the ideal, it is our 'natural state', and being fat is an unnatural and ugly symptom of a sick mind (sorry, mind, body and spirit); a physical manifestation of a mental defect to be healed, and proof of that healing would be sudden and permanent weight loss, if you'd just sign here...

What a comforting idea this would be if it were that simple, but buyer beware, this is the chocolate machine theory again: just put your money in the slot and eight inches of deep dark pleasure will plop into your receptacle, satisfaction guaranteed. We're being sold to again, girls. It sounds good; it even feels good couched in the love-language of the driven healer, but be sure, just as in the chocolate promise, it has no substance. We've been fleeced, we've been had, we've been taken to the cleaners already by so many others offering the final solution to wide hips. There isn't one, because being fat is not a psychological mistake, it's not a bad choice made by a traumatised mind, it is in fact an inherited quality usually common within a family, which comes, as with any birth gift, like having big feet or a large nose, or being short, or Polish, with challenges.

So although a lot of therapists of different persuasions have much to offer, and great strides can be made forward in your life by discovering and letting go old pain, when they nod at your hips and proclaim them curable, look deeper. And if they beckon to you and murmur, 'Come to my office twice a week for the next three years, cross my palm with copious amounts of silver, walk widdershins twice round the churchyard on a Wednesday, and don't step on the cracks in the pavement and maybe if you're very good you'll be healed', grab your handbag and run.

And when you have covered a fair distance, stop and ask yourself this: are you really convinced that life would so dramatically improve with less body fat? That all your problems would magically disappear with the fat cells? That thin people are happier, more fulfilled, have fewer problems and are at one with the earth?

Thigh size apart, we are all in this together; fat or thin we mostly face the same challenges. Personally I have got past blaming my buttocks for my misfortunes, in fact I have quite a peaceful mutual-admiration style relationship with my bottom. Oh lord, I hear that therapist's voice hissing in my ear, 'You're in denial – come to my office twice a week, bring the silver and on Wednesdays walk widdershins...' Not on your nelly. I'll take the high road and you take the low road and I'll be in Paradise before you, and make no mistake: this is not the temporary Paradise of briefly taking a smaller dress size, this is the Paradise of self-acceptance where everyone is an Angel irrespective of body size, the place of self-love and the constant celebration of the amazing diversity of human kind, the Paradise of true self value not dependent on other people's approval, of the joy of life for life's sake.

The Woman on the Finchley Omnibus

Liz Swinden

It was just an ordinary day. Getting on the bus to take me home from the tube station, I sat down on one of the sideways seats just inside. At the next stop I made room for a man to sit next to me. 'Why don't you move up a bit?' he said. Oh no, not again, I thought. He continued. 'Why don't you go on a diet so you can fit into the seats?'

Now everyone around us was listening. Would I just ignore him like a well-behaved, middle-aged woman or would I think of a smart reply that would blast him to kingdom come? What I actually said was, 'What makes you think you can go around being offensive to others?' He didn't reply and I got a cheer from one or two fellow travellers when I got off the bus.

I don't think I've ever been what you'd call small. Even as a baby, born at an average weight of 7lb 4oz, photographs of me show a solid, chunky, smiling, small person sitting on a cushion in a smocked dress with her dimpled little legs stuck straight out in front of her and clutching an apple in her hands – obviously much to the delight of her doting ma and pa.

Ma was a bit of a clothes horse, I realised many years later. Early photographs of her show a slim, leggy, flat-chested creature modelling clothes made for her by her mother, my lovely nanna who died when I was 12. Nanna was a dress-maker as well as a mannequin herself in the 1920s.

So my ma gave birth to this chubby little thing and then she fed her up and 'spoiled' her (well, she was an only child), and when sweets came off the ration she gave her too many of those, later dentists have confirmed. When I reached puberty and puppy fat, she turned tack and put me on a diet, promising lovely new clothes if I lost weight. I probably did too – Ma loved a challenge – although I really can't remember.

What I can remember is feeling fairly average. I knew I wasn't as knobbly and gawky as my friend Sandra or as gazelle-like as my friend Audrey, but I fitted into the grammar school uniform pretty well and I don't remember feeling out of place in my grey gym knickers and white aertex shirt with my initials embroidered in chain stitch. I didn't have a problem stripping off and running through the showers.

So why did my ma think there was something not quite right with her little girl? School photos show me as tall and solidly made but definitely nowhere near chubby and decidedly not fat. But the seeds of doubt about my acceptability as a female had been sown.

On a cut-price Costa Brava holiday with student friends in 1966, photographs show me in a pale blue bikini looking wonderfully curvy and absolutely okay, although I do remember being shouted at by some lads on the beach. Having sex was not a problem. I don't remember boyfriends saying I should be thinner, although in my first year at teacher training college, when I asked for the pill, I was told I would need to live on lettuce by the nice lady doctor at the Brook clinic. I mostly felt perfectly fine about my body.

In the early seventies, when feminism was taking hold and we were raising our consciousnesses all over the place, the Women's Therapy Centre held some workshops on eating disorders. I went along and joined a compulsive eaters' group, only to discover that I wasn't one and that the real issues weren't being addressed. Is it really better to be thin? What does the health research really show? Why does our society find it so hard to cope with fat women? How can a fat woman accept herself? These things are now being discussed, thank goodness.

As I entered marriage and became pregnant my weight began to creep up. I remember the consultant trying to make me admit to being diabetic as both kids were born at nine pounds plus. As a mother trying to feed small children, I began to see how important the connection was between food and feeling – how much women invest in the preparation of food and how children start to pick up messages about food very early on.

Since then I've got fatter and fatter. Now I'm definitely a big woman. I can't fasten the seat belts in some cars and I don't go into cafés or restaurants where the chairs are spindly designer models. I dress well but I can't shop at Marks & Spencer because they don't make anything in my size, except socks.

I try to love myself, body included, but it's not easy in a society that still condones making fun of us fat girls. What would some male TV presenters think of to say if Vanessa Feltz didn't exist, I sometimes wonder. Okay, if pushed, someone will admit that Dawn French is sexy and yes, more shops are stocking larger sizes in their ranges, but we've a long way to go before I will feel adequately reflected by the media.

My ma never saw me at the size I am now. She died ten years ago and I do miss her, even though if she was still here I suspect she'd be nagging me with a vengeance about my weight. When I lived in London and she lived in Manchester, whenever she saw me she'd make some remark about my appearance: 'Have you lost a bit of weight?' or some such. I don't blame her, though. Her only crime was to be born female and to be brought up, as we all are, to police each other's bodies as though it's the most natural thing in the world.

In 1988 one of the best things that happened to me was going to a meeting about fat and health. I was working in health promotion at the time and was getting fed up with all the usual talk about diet and exercise. Some women were there from the London Fat Women's group. They'd been meeting for some time supporting each other and working out a feminist analysis of fat oppression, but what they wanted to do was to put on a national conference. It'll be on a shoestring, they said, and so it proved, but we had journalists climbing up the walls of the London Women's Centre trying to get in.

Just being in the sauna that is the Women's Centre basement, surrounded entirely by women with ripe, luscious bodies, was something I won't forget in a hurry. Some of us went and did TV and radio interviews. I talked to John Humphrys and the late Brian Redhead on Radio 4's *Today*. We'd dropped a pebble in the pool and the ripples were simply enormous.

That's really how I got involved in the whole size acceptance movement. I'd always known somehow that there was something intrinsically wrong in trying to make yourself fit into society's preconceived idea of what a woman should look like. I also knew it would take a lot of effort and time to get things to change.

When I was working in health promotion, teachers used to phone me up and ask me how they could help girls they suspected of having anorexia or bulimia. I hadn't a clue. I didn't know much about eating disorders and quite honestly, at that point, I didn't have much sympathy for people who seemed to have so much control over what they ate that they could become as thin as Twiggy with no obvious effort. Just an instinctive reaction, I suppose. It seemed that if you were thin, you could not only get great clothes to fit, but you also got the sympathy of the medical establishment – unlike the 'obese' (horrid word). Later I learned it wasn't quite as simple as that.

Still, it got me thinking about how young women, and young men too, are socialised into thinking that body size is incredibly important. So important that at the age of about six, little girls are hugging their Barbie/Sindy dolls and using 'fat' as a term of abuse to their friends. Older ones are starving themselves to death in order to feel acceptable and those who *are* fat have their lives made hell by bullying.

I'd written a book for primary schools about sex education and my publishers were looking for new ideas. I said I wanted to do something on body image which would help teachers to raise the issues with young people in the classroom. Was it, I dared to hope, an idea whose time had come? Yes, I was told, go ahead. They liked the idea! So a colleague and I sat down and wrote it.

We looked at lots of different aspects of body image: exploring the concept of what is beautiful – Western society's Kate Moss or something else; physical perfection as an unattainable goal; insidious media images and how we can learn to deal with them; issues around gender – does it all start with Barbie and Action Man and end with anorexia or pumping iron?; attitudes to food – good foods/bad foods; the tyranny of dieting...

Let's face it, the list of things you want kids in school to start thinking about is a long one. But at least it's a start. Let's hope schools can squeeze it into the already overcrowded curriculum. Teachers know it's important to deal with these things, even if most of them are just as indoctrinated by the magazines, TV, and the beauty and fashion industries as the rest of us.

Now I'm middle-aged (eight years to retirement – what an appalling thought) and having night sweats. There are too many times when I seem about to forget my own name as well as other people's. It's an interesting time of life, that's all I'll say. Rather foolishly I'd thought that life would get easier or I'd get more tolerant. Not a bit of it. I still get angry when I see all the images of skinny little girls and so few representations of older, voluptuous, more mature bodies. What's wrong with middle-aged spread? If you don't see yourself reflected out there in the world, after a while you can be forgiven for thinking that you don't exist.

Last summer a friend and I were talking about the Carry On films and I pondered on whether anyone had written a book about Hattie Jacques. It turned out, after some research, that no one had. Amazing. A splendid actress, although usually typecast (unsurprisingly) in stereotypical roles. An icon of the British cinema and a wonderful role model for big women. So that's my next project and I know there's a publisher out there who will commission me to complete the research and write the book.

What keeps me going? My wonderful fat friends, and the thinner ones too, and the way we all support each other getting through this life. So back to the man and the woman on the Finchley omnibus. How did he get his bigoted views? Maybe a fat girl frightened him in the school playground when he was six. What are we to say or do to him to make him change his fat-phobic little mind? Sit on him perhaps?

To be frank I don't really know, except that whatever it is, we need to be honest and do whatever we do from our hearts. As a wonderful American woman called Alice Ansfield says, 'Think about the friends and supporters you have in your life. Let them know you love them. And think about whether there's some friend or family member it's time to approach with your truth and an open heart.' I want to tell what it is like to be judged by the shape and size of my body and if I do it with an open heart, I believe I will stand more chance of being heard and understood.

Heckling

Jo Brand

One aspect of my life as a comic which is always potentially life-threatening is the whole phenomenon of heckling.

As a fledgling comic, especially if you are a woman and a woman who doesn't look like a beautiful twig, you will have to face the fact that at some point, unless you only ply your trade at Sunday schools, you are going to get a mouthful from an audience member. Hecklers do not tend to discriminate between the sexes – they are quite happy to shout at anyone on stage – although there do tend to be some differences in the nature of the heckle. Women tend to get heckled mainly on some aspect of their appearance, whereas men will tend to be heckled about the content of their act. This isn't a hard and fast rule. Obviously, as a bloke, if you're unfortunate enough to be bald or have a huge nose, you will find your average heckler does not flounder about looking for a subtle yet devastating critique of you; he goes straight for the bleeding obvious.

My heckling experience has been, I would imagine, much the same as any other comic's. And as a fat person, I found out pretty sharpish that the majority of heckles were going to address my size, focusing on it to the extent that I occasionally feel moved to say to a heckler 'Do you honestly think I haven't heard that a million times before?'

In some ways, this makes life easier, because you are prepared. Hecklers do not spend hours at home practising their heckles, whereas comics have plenty of opportunity to try out put-downs. If you can come back with a personality destroying put-down the audience will love you and the heckler will slide down into his seat, smarting under the sneering gaze of his mates. All sounds so simple, doesn't it? If only life was like that.

First of all, hecklers are not clones and are as wide a variety as comics. Here are the main types:

The almost unconscious drunk

This heckler hardly even knows where he or she is. He/she shouts out utter rubbish at unpredictable intervals and cannot be silenced, even by the most clever of put-downs. This heckler must be thrown out or executed.

The aspiring comic

This heckler tries quite hard to be clever and funny and really thinks he is helping, when in fact he is just like an irritating little flea you have to keep constantly swatting. He will also come up to you at the end of the show and try and impress on you how much better he made the show go. Very annoying indeed.

The heckler with an axe to grind

This heckler has a specific political problem with your act and spends the entire show trying to turn your act into a debate like *Question Time*. A one-to-one argument doesn't go down well at a comedy performance, so it's best to silence them if you can.

The homicidal heckler

You can almost convince yourself that this heckler does actually want to kill you, so deeply offensive, obscene and terrifying is the depth of venom. Do not (as I considered once) attempt to attack them physically, as this is very unprofessional and a murder charge doesn't look great on your CV.

The heckler who is cleverer and funnier than you

This is every comic's worst nightmare and thankfully doesn't pop up very often. However, the solution is easy if you are prepared to humble yourself. Just acknowledge a funny heckle when you get one and don't get all flustered. It's going to happen, unless you are the funniest, most intelligent person in the world.

The other thing you have to bear in mind about comics dealing with hecklers is mood. Some days you feel great, other days you are as miserable as sin and you still have to make people laugh. If someone heckles you on a bad mood day, it is much easier to lose your temper or make a stupid decision. Once, suffering a suicidal combination of PMT and alcohol, I got into a 'discussion' with a Scots heckler about the history of England and Scotland, something I'd never even dream of doing normally.

I have managed to survive so far with a handful of put-downs, ranging from the quite sweet to the utterly obscene; for example 'I deliberately keep my weight up so a tosser like you doesn't fancy me' or 'Close your mouth or I'll sit on your face'. Many evenings, having used them all up in the first two minutes of my act, I've managed to fly by the seat of my pants and get off gracefully. I've been heckled off now and again, I've walked off now and again and, on one occasion, I've dissolved into tears like a true Barbara Cartland heroine. Hecklers can be hurtful, but no worse, on the whole, than your average building site neanderthal.

Looking like you don't give a toss is ultimately your greatest weapon and I use this off stage as well. People always tell me I look so confident on stage when I'm tackling a heckler. Little do they know that in my head I am planning a very painful torture or having a little girlie sniffle.

Lesbian at Large

Esther D Rothblum

Several years ago, I was interviewed by a feminist sociologist for a study of 'successful fat women'. At the end of the interview, she asked me whether, if I could live my life over again, I would prefer to be heterosexual. I responded that I loved being a lesbian; I would be seriously depressed if I ever became heterosexual. She then asked if I could live my life over again as a thin woman, would I do so? Absolutely, I answered.

Being fat and being lesbian have played different roles in my life. But it is difficult to view my weight and my sexual orientation as separate from other aspects of myself. I am also white, Jewish, able-bodied, an immigrant living in the USA, and 44 years old. As a psychologist and a university professor, I have conducted research, separately, about lesbians and about fat women, and here too the research has diverged. Whereas it has become 'mainstream' to be a lesbian researcher, it is quite controversial still to conduct research about fat women, especially since I too am a member of this group.

I grew up in an upper-middle class family. My father was a diplomat and I spent my childhood years in Yugoslavia, Spain, Brazil, Nigeria and Austria. Like most diplomatic families, mine was anxious to keep up appearances.

Beginning when I was four years old, my father's annual holiday letter to friends and colleagues expressed dismay over my weight. In fact, old photographs show me to be average weight until age eight, when I became a chubby child. Now my weight and appearance dominated family discussions. I was sure that it was the first thing people noticed about me.

In my Nigerian elementary school, we all collected stamps to send to an agency that cured lepers. My teacher, Mrs Uzochuko, had harsh words for the student who didn't bring in an allotment of old postage stamps. Once a term she would send the packet of stamps off and then fume when the expected thank you letter didn't arrive immediately. Sooner or later the agency would send the letter along with a bag of candy. Then Mrs Uzochuko would walk through the classroom, stopping to place one sweet on each child's desk – except for the children she felt were too fat to eat sweets. I sat drowning in shame while Mrs Uzochuko told Jane Graham, Lami Coker and Nwabwazi Wachuko that fat children shouldn't eat sweets, waiting for my own public shaming. But I got a sweet. At the time I thought it was because I was the teacher's pet, but now I think I simply wasn't as fat as the other students.

Unlike the way my weight was counted and noted, thankfully, perhaps, I had no comparable way of expressing my lesbianism. I can remember being attracted to girls since the age of four, and fantasising about the girls who sat next to me on the school bus when I was six. These feelings were clearly erotic, not just memories of close affection. Being attracted to other girls was easy; my parents approved of close friendships and allowed me to spend the night with these friends. In contrast, had I been attracted to boys, there would have been general alarm. Nor did I see my weight as an impediment in developing these friendships.

I remember precisely when I became a fat activist. Now as an adult I was in love with a woman who I will call Jay. Jay wore a size six but worried about her weight – she was the heaviest in a very, very thin family. Jay was not sexually or romantically interested in me, but instead she went through a number of lovers while spending a lot of time with me. I could handle it when her lovers were male, but became devastated when I saw her become attracted to a woman. This new woman in Jay's life seemed a mirror image of me – same height, similar hair, about the same age, comparable sense of humour, similar occupation – but she was average weight. It was proof to me that I was everything Jay wanted in a woman except for my weight. It was also one of the only ways that being lesbian and being fat converged for me; my parents had always said that if I failed to become thin I would 'never marry'.

So I toyed with the idea of losing weight, becoming the kind of woman that Jay would find attractive. I knew that diets in women's magazines were unsound, probably just the editor's notion of something to insert between the obligatory ads for weight-loss products. I went to the psychological literature, where clinical researchers randomly assigned fat women to various treatment groups. In a typical study, women might be part of either Treatment A (say, exercise) or Treatment B (perhaps a very low calorie diet) or Treatment A + B that combined the two. A fourth group of women would be assigned to a waiting list control group that received no 'treatment' at all. I even had first-hand knowledge of this kind of research study, as in graduate school I had helped out a friend conduct her dissertation on weight loss groups.

But now, for the first time, I was looking at this kind of published research article with an eye to finding the ideal diet. I was appalled at how little weight the women really lost and how much they regained, regardless of which 'treatment' they received. A year after the studies had ended, the women were usually enticed to come back for one final 'weigh-in'. At that point, no one had maintained much weight loss and were generally no different from the women who had been on the waiting list. So that was the end of my having any thoughts about dieting and the beginning of my fat activism.

During a week of spring vacation in the 1980s I wrote a lengthy review article about the flaws in the research on women and weight, which I titled *Women and Weight: Fad and*

Fiction. Submitting an article to an academic journal is done one journal at a time; one can't just send it out to a dozen editors and wait to see which ones reply. I got so many rejections that I now have a slide show of some of the most blatant, hostile comments. But each time my article was returned I immediately sent it off to another journal. Two years and many rejections later, my article was finally accepted for publication. The managing editor of the journal in which the article finally appeared wrote to say that this article 'is certainly one of the most outstanding pieces we have published in the *Journal of Psychology* during my time as managing editor'. Such are the vagaries of journal publishing!

At the same time, I was conducting research on lesbian issues. Here, in contrast, editors were eager to accept whatever I submitted. I once even had three editors all vying to publish the same study (about lesbian sex at menopause), which was based on a smaller sample and used a less stringent methodology than any one of my studies on weight. In fact, were I not conducting research on lesbians, with corresponding acceptances, I would have thought that my research on weight was somehow flawed.

In many ways, getting *Women and Weight: Fad and Fiction* published gave me (and the colleagues and students who collaborated) the self-confidence to proceed with a series of research studies. We conducted two studies about weight and employment discrimination. One asked members of NAAFA (the National Association to Advance Fat Acceptance) about their own experiences of weight-related employment discrimination and also about employment-related victimisation (such as being told in school not to go on to university because of their weight, or urged into school or university programmes that would be less affected by their weight). In the second study, undergraduate students were asked to evaluate a job résumé of a woman weighing 150lbs. The results were disturbing. The students gave this woman a low rating on her likeability as a co-worker, and for her supervisory potential, self-discipline, professional appearance, personal hygiene and ability to do a physically strenuous job. However, when the students evaluated the identical résumé, with the weight changed to 120lbs, they gave it a much higher rating.

One of the issues that interested me about the employment experiences of fat people was whether a lifetime of social rejection denied them the opportunities to develop social skills. We examined this in two separate studies about weight and social skills. We asked fat and thin women to converse with someone over the telephone, so that no one would know that the study focused on weight. Then we audiotaped the telephone conversations and asked raters to evaluate the women's social skills. In the first study, university under-graduates rated the audiotapes of the fat women as less likeable, less socially skilled, and less physically attractive than the audiotapes of the average weight women, without knowing which was which. So it would seem that fat women don't have the same social skills as thin women.

However, those who are members of oppressed groups often learn to compensate for their stigmatised condition. So in the second study, fat and thin women had a telephone conversation with a 'telephone partner' whom they could not see, but we told some of them that their telephone partner could see them over the video monitor. When the fat women thought they *could* be seen by their telephone partners, they did something to improve their social skills and these were rated more highly by the evaluators. When the fat women thought they could not be seen, they did not 'compensate' in this way and received lower ratings on social skills.

We found that fat women are rated lower on social skills by strangers, particularly when the women can't be seen and thus weight should not be an issue. So a lifetime of prejudice does affect how we behave in the world. However, fat women have learned to compensate for this stigmatised condition so we do improve how we are rated when we think our weight is apparent. However, fat women are rated no differently than thin women on social skills by people such as friends and colleagues, who know them well – when the women know they are accepted and can perhaps relax. Possibly the women in the first study were protecting themselves from rejection, which they felt would happen if they got the job and met the employer.

Wanting to find out how lesbians are affected by the stigma of weight, I wrote a review article in which I looked at several factors that might account for how physical appearance is related to sexual orientation. Lesbians are not immune from societal pressures to be attractive, though they may be *less* influenced by appearance norms since they do not interact sexually with men. But the lesbian community has its own norms for appearance, and these change over time and across region. The process of 'coming out' involves being recognised by and recognising other lesbians. The dominant culture has negative attitudes towards lesbians, including perceptions of lesbians' appearance. And multicultural lesbians may be affected by appearance norms from the lesbian and dominant groups, as well as other minority groups.

To examine some of these issues, I conducted a study that compared lesbians, gay men, and heterosexual women and men on weight, dieting, preoccupation with weight, and exercise activity. Heterosexual women and gay men (that is, people who are in relationships with men) reported wanting to weigh less and were more preoccupied with weight than were lesbians or heterosexual men (that is, people who are in relationships with women). However, gender was on the whole more significant than sexual orientation, with both lesbians and heterosexual women reporting greater concern with weight, more body dissatisfaction, and greater frequency of dieting than did gay or heterosexual men. The results show that both lesbians and heterosexual women are influenced by cultural pressures to be thin, but these pressures may be greater for heterosexual women.

People in the US are so obsessed with slimness and have

such negative attitudes towards fatness, that we are not aware of our cultural isolation regarding these views and we cannot understand how anyone could view fatness positively. In order to compare US statistics with those of another Western nation, I spent two summers in Australia researching attitudes about weight. As in the US, weight was a much greater issue for women in Australia, who felt more overweight, dieted more, expressed more body self-consciousness, and reported that weight had interfered more with social activities, than did men. However, Australian college students were *less* likely to be dieting, less concerned with their weight and less self-conscious about their bodies than were comparable students in the US.

Similarly, when we compared students in the US to those at a university in Ghana in West Africa, we found the US students more likely to diet, and more preoccupied with thinness in themselves and in other people. But once again, weight was more of an issue for women (across nationality) than for men.

I am intrigued (and dismayed, as a fat woman myself) about the fact that there are so few political organisations for fat people. Why is this so? Thinness is one of the major criteria in determining physical attractiveness in the US. It is difficult for women to violate appearance norms – they are not trivial. However, fat people, particularly women, tend to be poor in the US, and thus have little political power. And fat people are blamed for their weight – most people believe that diets are effective if the dieter has 'willpower'. Since weight loss is rarely permanent, it would seem important to change people's attitudes about the *lack* of control that they – and others – have over body weight.

It is now more than a decade since my first research on weight appeared in print. And since then I have been cited in newspapers and magazines in the US and Britain. Slowly, painfully, the media are beginning to realise that diets don't work and that fat people suffer prejudice and discrimination in the US. I am finding journalists (and the general public) a bit more aware of the issues, a bit less likely to make hostile remarks about fat people.

Still, I find the weight research area exhausting, even with the small steps that have been made. When I hear an anti-lesbian remark, I can expect sympathy from other lesbians. There is no comparable expectation of empathy when I experience hostile anti-fat comments.

But I have found that life gets better as I age. It is easier to be a fat woman in my forties than a close-to-average weight child or a chubby adolescent. I have the 'weight' of my professional identity to fall back on and I have a lot of economic privilege. I also love my body, and I think this helps other people appreciate it. And I have found a few fat-affirmative allies, some of them in surprising places . . .

Full Fat

Jane Goddard Carter

The fat person can sometimes be left wondering about the motivation and integrity of friends. Is that person I share jolly girly gossips with a real friend? Or is she a patronising, co-dependent manipulator who offers her brand of friendship only if I play the role she has decided I should play, without deviation?

When I was asked to write this piece I told a particular friend, 'I've been asked to contribute to an anthology of writings by fat women, celebrating our lives as fat women.' My friend responded in shrill, whiny tones 'Ohhh dear Jane! I really don't think you should do it, because I don't think of you in *that* way.' She went on and on, loading my ears with her conciliatory apologies for me being me; telling me in her clumsy way that her opinion of me (a patronising denial of all that I actually am) was more valid than any opinion I might hold of my own. I reached for a pen and drew a heavy line through her name on my Christmas and birthday list. I drew the type of line that makes me wonder if a pen is the right weapon for me to be wielding. On reflection a pen is just the right weapon to use, and I will show you why.

For too long, far too long, big fat women and the presence we offer to the world have been shaped by the opinions of others: others who are not big and not fat. We are expected to conform to the stereotype that the prejudiced, collective mind dictates for us. And the saddest part of this is that it is women, more often than not, who are the fat woman's worst enemy.

I look around me and I see fat folks of all ages, shapes, sizes, persuasion and gender, wearing their bodies as burdens to be loathed by themselves and others; weighed down, not just by the physical discomfort of being very fat, but by the disgust and distaste of our society. I see fat friends slumped beneath rounded shoulders − backs aching, not filling their bodies or brains with enough oxygen to vitalise their size. I want to shout, 'Walk tall, breathe, fill your lungs, fill your brains with oxygen, feed yourselves, feed your spirits!' But I too have been in that horrid state where I perceived my body as a stifling burden. I know how deaf with despair it is possible to be to suggestions that doing anything at all would enable my spirit to live a life worth living. But no more folks, no more.

I am big by biological design. I have a wide, tall body, built for strenuous activity. It makes sense to me to fill that body with my presence. It's a little like the difference between those who can really 'wear' a hat and those who can't, who are worn by the hat. It has nothing to do with physical appearance but everything to do with the confidence of the wearer.

I am put in mind of a recent evening at a comedy gig. The headline act was a sometime half of a BBC launch series for alternative comedians. Once he was a beautiful, pale, gothic lovely, swathed in velvet as he delivered his sad and cynical comic tales of life, love, despair and football. Three years, one miserable novel, much less success than his one-time laddish comedy partner, later, he turned up on tour. He shambled out on stage, lager in hand, pasty-faced, lank, paunchy and clad in beer-stained khaki fatigues. He stood in front of the microphone and delivered his act with little enthusiasm, effort or style. This one-time hero of comedy had abandoned all pretence of being alive. He had become fat and looked and sounded as if he had given up. The audience laughed, but it sounded like dutiful, disappointed laughter.

How unlike the laughter that greeted his support act. The support act had bounced on to the stage, greeting his audience with 'Oh dear, they've sent us a fat lad!' He was fat, very fat, but he filled his body, clothes and the theatre with vibrant presence, with far more oomph than gothic sad boy. He dressed to accentuate his size for dramatic effect. He was stylish, bright and bursting with energy. He worked hard for his laughs, very hard. He made some references to his size, but this was not the backbone of his act, just the accent. He cleverly niggled at the prejudices held against the fat without resorting to the self-deprecating, undignified 'I'll slag myself off before you get a chance to' throwaway, collusive lines that encourage prejudice. Because he acknowledged the way he was, that evening he was funnier than the headline act. He was comfortable with himself, he wasn't pretending to be thin, he was honest and his honesty and confidence gave him freedom.

My ex-friend on the phone wanted me to be dishonest with myself. She is uncomfortable when I refer to my size, because she herself is uncomfortable around fat. Moreover she is terrified of it. She wants all fat people to be cowed, beaten and sad, to feel as if they are living inside the enemy. To be constantly trying to alter, restrict and distort themselves into an unattainable mode of behaviour and physical state. My confidence in being me, perhaps, made her aware of how precarious her own confidence is.

Showing confidence in inhabiting the big, fat body is rare. Being confident in our size requires more energy and bravery than many people can muster. When we have that confidence we shine. We shine more brightly than any digitally enhanced, gaunt, pubescent coathanger who may gaze at us from every billboard or magazine page. When we arrive, we arrive big time. We can be loud, shy or just plain ordinary, but we are there, like it or not. So why not be as big as we are? Why live in a perpetual state of apology? I enjoy being big. I will not despise parts of me that wobble, crease or fold, just because I am told to. I will show my strength, my substance.

One area of life for the fat woman in our society that is often the cause of desperate sighs and groans, is fashion. Money and prejudice frequently decree that we, with our wonderful variety of sensual shapes, should be excluded from expressing ourselves through the medium of attire. Sadly, even the fat women who work in fat fashion shops collude with those who would stifle our expression, encouraging us to be grateful for the shapeless, poorly made Crimplene tents that are offered in lieu of style and quality. So what do I do about it? Well, every time I go into a shop and can't find what I want to wear, I gripe very loudly about it, especially in the hearing of other customers. If I am offered conciliatory explanations for the lack of size range I treat the assistants to a little civil rights polemic, and the shop loses a customer and the money that customer brings. Sometimes I will phone the head of design and let her know why the efforts she and her team are making are simply not good enough. No one is going to tell me what I should wear and expect to get away with it. If I want to wear a tight red velvet Lycra body suit, then I damn well will. What is more, I'll look more stylish and beautiful than anyone else within a five-mile radius to boot. Sure, I will attract a lot of attention by doing so, and some of it will be offensive, but I am determined to be seen, to be visible. Being fat and visible is a challenge, one I am definitely up to. If I am honest, I enjoy it.

When you are physically bigger than most of those around you, people do get out of your way. On the street, in shops, in cinemas, theatres, buses, anywhere. A certain amount of fun can be had because of it. I don't care if the skinny young woman (size eight, but wants to be a size six) occupying the window seat on the train, plasters herself against the grubby glass to avoid being squashed or tainted by my fatness – no indeed! I shall sit next to her, even if the rest of the carriage is full of nothing but tumbleweeds and an eerie wind. Even if several handsomely constructed, tastefully pierced, oiled up Nubian gentlemen implore me to sit upon lovingly prepared satin cushions in my own special carriage – I will sit next to her. Why? Because her kind have terrorised my kind with this society's brand of oppression for long enough. They would just love my kind to disappear. But obviously we are not going to. Never a day passes without some mention in the media of the growing percentage of our population who are fat. So here I am – in your face. If I am feeling really mean, I might just engage her in a pleasant conversation. One that she – very reluctantly – will find herself delighted by, wanting more of in fact. If I have had a really bad day (and lordy sometimes there are enough of those!) and I want some further entertainment, I might just eat some chocolate in front of her. Perhaps I'll even offer her some, delighting in her discomfort, her embarrassment. For her, there is no such thing as the simple, sensuous pleasure of chocolate, oh no. Not only does it come in a box marked guilt and fear, it is iced with the shame of being offered by and accepted from a fat person.

So where does this bolshy attitude to living in a big fat body come from? My endurance is born out of adversity; my vigour, from a lifelong battle with the prejudice and blinkered perception that most fat people encounter.

The real breakthrough came when I decided that life was too short to be constantly giving in to the command from the media and peers of 'Sod off, you are fat, ergo you are no good.' I started to get fit, very fit. I had always been pretty active and outward bound, but forever bowing to the yap of the shocked and disapproving bicycles lagging at my heels. If I dared to show my physical prowess, especially if I could do something better than they, I would want to hide that achievement away, where it wouldn't attract the spite of jealous detractors. But no more, sisters, no more! Now, I boldly dance, leap, lift and astound. I endure. I have stamina and strength. I have agility and elegance. I have style – big dramatic hair, clothes, a rhythmic gait, expansive gestures. I shine, I really do. Whenever and wherever I can, I live it to the full. I use the shape of my body and the shape of my mind to be lively, sharp and sensuous.

I rather revel in shock and surprise – they are useful tools in irritating bigots. A few years ago I took up belly dancing.

Surprise, surprise! I found that I was pretty good at it. Many teachers of this art are the skinny, old hippy has-been club, you know the type – went to Morocco in the late sixties, picked up on the tribal woman vibe, blanked out the fact that the women whose culture they were stealing were good, broadhipped wobblers. They then came back to this country with a licence to print money and, perhaps unwittingly, perpetuate prejudice. In their dance classes, they hold forth about 'accepting and celebrating the whole woman, within and without', but unfortunately their particular brand of acceptance and celebration doesn't include fat women, within, without or whatever. So when I turn up with my competent basic repertoire of shimmies, wiggles and walks, as good as their most esteemed (but skinny) teacher's pet, I am treated to the usual patronising 'Oh Jane, you do dance well for...' I just love to finish the sentence: 'For what? A fat bird?' Yes, I do dance well, certainly not in spite of my size, but because of it. Belly dancing requires a belly and a good weighty arse. I have got both, nice ones too! I love it when a shimmy takes on a life of its own: it looks and feels wonderful. Shock and surprise on the faces of others are rewards as well.

Riding horses attracts similar kinds of jealous response. I have been riding since I was three years old. That is a total of 35 years of experience, 35 years of fairly serious study and practice of the art. No, I am not perfect, far from it. But if I am seen to be getting the right sort of movement out of a difficult horse, I occasionally hear bitchy women say, 'She's only getting it right because she has so much weight, so much force to use.' No! I get it right simply because I know my body well, I know how to use it, to regulate its strength. I don't need to use force – my gravitas, my balance and my brain get the result I want.

When scrawny doctors take my blood pressure or measure my cholesterol, I merrily challenge their surprise that I am fitter than they. I dance from the surgery, leaving jaws dropped to the floor, aghast that I should dare to affront their expectations. Mentally I suggest that they swivel upon my proffered middle finger, indulging my gleeful compulsion to confront and break down prejudice.

I believe that fat women probably have a more thorough awareness and knowledge of their bodies than their thinner sisters, because they are reminded of their bodies at every moment of their lives. Yes, through the impoliteness of society, but also by the fat body itself. The undulating folds of the fat body wobble and shimmy of their own accord, whatever you do. So why spend your life hating what is there? Many fat women pretend they aren't fat. They bind and truss themselves up in corsets, fooling no one, least of all themselves. What a waste of energy! The physical voice of the fat body will always be whispering away in your ear – 'Here I am, folding, bulging and wiggling away!' – so why not get to know that voice? It isn't your enemy; it is you. Don't hate your fat self. That way lies misery.

It occurs to me that the practice of social exclusion is a dangerous specialisation, a monoculture. In evolutionary terms, diversity is healthier. Prejudice is a great stifler of human potential – it leads to depravation; depravation of experience and the opportunity to live life to the full. In the new century, in the pursuit of humaneness, surely we should be delighting in the variety of human form, and more importantly, perpetuating it – for our survival.

I haven't always been like this and on some days my bravado deserts me. I can feel outflanked by a world where my size dictates what work I am offered, how seriously I am taken, how respectfully I am treated. Some days the effort is too great. There are days when I don't want to be noticed. These are the days when plain rudeness gets to me, when I want to slap the skinny cow who tells me I would look prettier and less fat if I grew my fringe longer. Days when I want to hurl abuse at the fat, jealous, insecure friend who tells me that I should dress in loose clothes as it is more flattering to the fuller figure. Days when I dress down, days when I just want to be the same as everybody else. But as I get older those days are fewer. Being big has made me examine myself closely, perhaps in too much detail: 'Did it turn out that way because I am fat, or just because I am me?' Too much of that type of in-depth analysis can bog you down in a mire of ambiguity and inaction. But at the end of the day I believe I am better fat and knowing myself, than thin without a clue.

With so much of our media saying 'Yeeeuch! it's a fat bird – sod off, ugly' it is sometimes forgotten that there is anyone out there who admires our bodies. It is a secret that doesn't often get out. Oh yes – my ample bosomyness is often appreciated. But, bad news for all those boys who think I'll be grateful for any sexual attention I can get – I have a choice, and I can choose not to be free with my assets. No, boys, just because I am big, it doesn't mean I am your mammy – oh no. You must appreciate me as I am, a big, vibrant, fleshy sun. Have me as a vast and pleasant treat only. Be grateful. Be polite and most of all be careful. This gentle, juicy gravitas that comforts and indulges your wildest desires can, if she is displeased or discovers motives she doesn't wholly approve of, turn and squash your tiny frame to so much (so little) dust.

There is a light at the end of the tunnel. After so many years of atrocious oppression, some sections of our culture are now able to recognise and tolerate, if not necessarily acknowledge and accept, the myriad voices of the marginalised: of the female, black, gay, lesbian, disabled, transvestite and transsexual etc. Even if these voices are not always respectfully accommodated into our actual behaviour or truly listened to, they are still, on occasion, heard. Being heard is the important thing. It is one of the first steps of learning. Once society is able to abandon its deafness, once it can hear, it can then learn to listen, absorb, change its attitude and its behaviour.

These days it is possible to turn on the television or radio and daily find at least one programme devoted to 'Fat' – be it an exploitative, confessional chat show or an arrogant, institutionally driven, finger-wagging lecture on the perils of living the life of lard. Much of the output has the taint of the freakshow. Nevertheless, it is exposure for the voice of the fat. At the same time, humming around in the air like an echo hell-bent on sabotage, is the complaining voice of some of those involved in the apologetically named Fat Acceptance Movement, devaluing this exposure. I say, don't decry it, feed it, add to it, get inside it, sway it gently in the direction you want.

In the early days of any civil rights movement, the first language the oppressor uses to describe what it has heard, is its own. I really believe that the time will come when the oppressor will consider what it has heard, and will want to talk back to us. Then we'll have the breakthrough. To communicate effectively, a respectful language will have to be used, and best of all, we will be the ones who set the terms and conditions. For so long, we have been hidden away, shamefully swathed in unfashionable, ugly clothes or ghettoised into roles that have little to do with our actual selves. I hope that I live long enough to see the day when the voice of fat experience, the voice that sings of its joys and triumphs, not just its misery and defeat, is really listened to, incorporated into everyday life and accorded the validity and respect it deserves.

In another 2000 years' time I should quite like to be preserved as a sophisticated, animatronic exhibit in some millennial museum, celebrating the diversity of life on this planet. What tales would I tell? Would I sit submissively, unattractively dressed in a quasi-multicultural print, Crimplene tent dress, gently ululating and droning my way through dull, historical texts of mild, earthy femaleness – taking it all a bit too seriously and frightening the visiting school children? No bloody way. I'll be sitting astride a vast, black, spiky maned horse. I'll be dressed in the tight black leather of the all-powerful, belly-dancing warrior woman proudly showing my strength, my magnitude. One hand would wield an elegant, wind-rippled battle pennant proclaiming 'Magna In Aeternum'. Beneath the hooves of the horse would lie the broken bodies of the tiny – the tiny of mind that is.

A Fine Big Woman

Joanne Simms

I am a fine big woman. I had the proof, if proof I needed, one night in the Glenelg Inn, having a drink with Jimmy Watt.

While I was standing at the bar an amiable old drunk leaned over from his stool and slapped me swiftly on the bottom, bit my upper arm and said admiringly: 'My, Jimmy, but she's a fine big woman.'

'Hey, Jimmy, that bloke's just bitten me!'

'You're a big girl, you can take care of yourself.' He turned back to his dram and talk of boats and fishing. Good beer and food, yes, but the Glenelg has never been, nor will ever evolve into, a hotbed of chivalry.

Given my size 18 I am a big woman, if womanhood is to be measured by fashion and not by nature. I would argue that I am a woman-sized woman, if the evidence of the women who have gone before me and can be seen in art galleries and museums is anything to go by. The likes of today's stick-thin, boy-girl, woman-child models have never before been considered a vision of beauty; rather they would be tucked away in a corner of some allegorical Biblical scene to represent famine and despair.

The message sent out by the pictures of women today is confusing, both sexually and physically. How are big women and large teenagers supposed to feel good about themselves when the current ideal is for skinny waifs?

I know this is a well-travelled point of view. It has been argued far better elsewhere, and must be so boring for so many blasé people, but please consider this: there is something terribly wrong, if not slightly obscene, about a society which tells its young women that to look beautiful, fashionable and desirable, they must be heroin thin.

At the same time this same society devotes an increasing amount of its media to food and cookery programmes and pays only lip service to the plight of those nations where people die through war, famine and irredeemable national debt.

During my twenties and thirties I admit that I succumbed to the monstrous pressure put on women to conform to the fashion industry's desire for women to stay forever young and androgynous. I dieted, joined Weight Watchers and my scales yo-yoed.

Oh yes, that desperate desire for approval, that hellish feeling of inadequacy.

Young men I went out with chose me and then, in the age-old power-dance between men and women, set about changing me into what they thought I should be and therefore what I should want to be. This prompts the question, if I was not what you wanted, why want me in the first place? But then that can be found at the source of all kinds of wonderful problems and tangles we get ourselves into as we stumble through life. And at the time, twit that I was, I was willing to oblige. Ever wished you could travel backwards through time and space and give yourself a bloody good talking to?

As I dropped two stone at Weight Watchers the man I was with suggested buying me a gold chain for my waist and having it fastened so that I'd know if I were getting too big. Back then I thought it was so romantic. Now, over 20 years on, I could think sick, pervert, control-freak; but all I can do is laugh out loud and think yuck.

Then there was the wonderful, kind, gentle thinker who coaxed me into joining him in his other passion, running. His life was dedicated to marathons, fell running and training every day whether injured or ill. We would go to the Lake

District and I would walk up fells he had planned for me, my two to his five or six. He would get our routes to cross at lunch, or I'd reach a summit and find a love letter or course changes wrapped round a piece of Kendal Mint cake. He fell in love with a fat, mumsy woman who loved him very much, but he wanted to change me into something I wasn't. I even ran 10K races, in a kind of cotton iron-lung sports bra, wondering what was going to burst first, my left knee or my heart.

I decided it had to end when he proudly showed me his last toenail, which had fallen off that morning. In the macho world of hard running its loss proved something. As the sad, brown, sickening crisp sat proudly in the palm of his hand, in an entrance hall which always had a background aroma of well-used running shoes and the sheep-shit they'd run through, I knew I had to leave. I broke his heart; it broke my heart, but better to amputate before the rot sets in.

Why the hell do I only seem to attract sporty men who then want me to join them? There was a parachutist but that ended after a month. On my thirty-ninth birthday I met a young ski-instructor with buttocks so hard you could break a fingernail on them, a café-au-lait tan, Sean Connery accent and blue eyes to die for. I could see the signs; he started talking about nursery slopes. I told him politely and tactfully that I wasn't interested and it worried friends a great deal that I wasn't, but I wasn't. He still keeps vaguely in touch and pops in to see me every year between summers canoeing and winters skiing. Oh the joy of being old enough to know your own mind. Ten or fifteen years ago I'd have been half-drowned or frostbitten in no time.

Back then, I probably verged on bulimic. The day I realised I was contemplating going into the lavatory to stick my fingers down my throat I frightened myself enough to decide the whole game could go to hell.

My weight and I settled down over a couple of years to a comfortable shape and size that both my body and I are happy with. Perhaps again it is something to do with age and the gaining of some measure of maturity and confidence in yourself. When you become your own woman, you become your own natural shape and size.

I am built for comfort not speed, I tell the men in my life these days.

'Come over here and let's get comfy then,' is the usual reply.

But recently I have had a very uncomfortable time of it when I lost weight through illness. What I thought was a niggle from a rib broken in a riding accident turned out to be gallstones. Overnight my weight dropped and with it went my self-image and a large dollop of confidence.

My gall bladder was removed and the stones offered to me in a little bottle to take home as a souvenir. The nurse sounded a bit huffy when I refused: 'Don't you want them, then?'

'I thought the whole idea was that I came in here and got rid of them, love.'

I came out of hospital 12 pounds lighter and the weight kept falling, as my body told me it preferred a low-fat diet. I could only look on in despair as my lovely round bosom disappeared, so clothes hung on me and waistbands slipped towards my belly button.

My pretty lace 38D bras could have pleats put in them. I was going straight up and down. I could only look in horror as the shape that I was as a sickly child slowly emerged; my eyes started to look too big for my face, just like in old family photographs.

I felt my femininity was dissolving. I said to a woman at work that I'd lost just over a stone in six months; I was saying it in despair, she thought I was saying it in triumph and asked how I'd done it because she'd like to lose a bit of weight, too.

At one stage the skin seemed to be hanging on me, looking, I thought, like crepe paper. I just sat on the edge of my bed and cried.

This was all stupid really, a form of vanity, I kept telling myself. How many times have I lectured my fellow woman on accepting her natural shape? Come on, get a grip, I would scold myself as the bathroom scales confirmed what the mirror kept telling me.

It was time for the post-operative me to take a dose of the medicine I was always dishing out while standing on my own personal soap box and going on at women complaining about their weight. If nature said that I was going to lose weight, I should just shut up and accept it.

You are the shape you are; love it.

I might have had to love it, but I didn't have to put up with it! I went out to investigate the purchase of a padded bra for the first time in my life.

In forty-odd years I have hugged a lot of people to my bosom, in moments of passion or comfort or reassurance. Just then I needed some reassurance of my own, even if it was only going to be courtesy of Gossard.

Since the dark days of 36C and foam filling, the weight has been coming back slowly. When the lady in the Marks & Spencer bra fitting department put her tape measure down and announced 'thirty-eight C, dear' I don't think I had felt so good since I passed my driving test.

I know: I go on and on about the sexual and social politics of weight. But recent events have shown me that when it comes to how I feel about how I look I am just as guilty as the poor sods who starve themselves and stick their fingers down their throats, only in reverse.

'You've got your wiggle back,' an old friend told me at a party.

'My what?'

'You know, your wiggle in your . . .' he started to blush, bless him. I actually know a man who is heading for 55 years old and he still blushes.

'My where?'

By now he was crimson: 'Never mind where. It's just back.'

It's back all right, and it's a damned fine big one.

Jeans, Jumpers and Clingy Tops

Gladeana McMahon

I happened into the world a month early after my mother was knocked down on a zebra crossing in a hit and run incident. The birth was difficult and I popped out weighing just over three pounds, leaving a somewhat exhausted mother to recuperate. In 1954 a three-pound baby was cause for concern. The nursing staff called me 'the shrimp' and were all impressed by my will to survive. My mother always took great pride in telling me how they backed a horse named 'Never Say Die' – the horse won and I survived. Six months after leaving the hospital, on one of her daily shopping expeditions she met the ward Sister who was totally amazed at just how much I had grown.

From the photographs I have of myself as a baby I seemed to continue to grow in all directions and soon became a chubby toddler. I was an inquisitive child and couldn't wait to start school. My mother learned to take an alternative route to the one which went past our local school as I would ask (in the alarmingly repetitive way that only children can) why I couldn't go to school *now* every time we passed the school gate. The day came for me to go to school and I was full of excitement. I wanted to look my best and I remember trying on many different outfits before settling on the one I felt presented me at my best. Sadly, school fell far short of my expectations. So much so that I told my mother the following Monday that I had 'tried school for a week' and, as I did not like it, would not be returning. From hanging on to the railings in a desperate bid to get in, I now hung on to the same railings in an equally desperate bid to keep out. I lost the battle and many years of misery began.

Although an intelligent child, I could not take to school. It seemed to me that the questions I wanted answered never were. During my time at primary school I began to recognise I was different from the other children. True, I was a person of colour at a time when there were fewer children of non-white extraction. My Muslim father came from Bangladesh, and my Jewish mother came from the North of England. (It is believed that her ancestors came from Russia. However, I've never been able to find out the whole story as the impact of anti-Semitism proved too great for my grandparents and they distanced themselves from their cultural origins, changed names and sent their children to chapel.) Being called a 'coffee coloured wog' when I was eight was the first but not the last racist comment I remember. However, it was not the colour of my skin or my cultural origins which caused me to feel different.

I began to realise I was larger than other children. At first the realisation meant very little. But as time went by and I began to compare myself, feelings of alienation took root. By the time I was ten I was indeed a 'big girl'. So big that at one of the regular medical checks by the school doctor my mother was called in to talk about my weight. My mother was enraged and made no bones about telling the doctor that big was healthy. The fact that she and the majority of women in our family were also large may have contributed to my mother's attitude. Nothing further happened and I graduated to my secondary school. Having failed my eleven plus I did not get a place at the prestigious grammar school my parents wanted me to attend but went to a local comprehensive instead.

Ackland Burghley became my home for the next five years. The first year brought academic acclaim but sadly it went downhill after that. I could not see much sense in the education being offered, struggled with maths (even with the help of a private tutor) and preferred to spend my time doing art, drama and music. It was at this comprehensive that the bullying began in earnest. I weighed ten stone. It seemed to me my school uniform never really fitted and that all the other girls left school at the end of the day as neat and tidy as they began, while I always looked as if I had been pulled backwards through the proverbial hedge.

Looking back I can see how I was a prime candidate for bullying. I was fat, wore glasses, was a different colour, did not play sport, was easily upset and preferred the teachers to many of the pupils. While the bullying increased from name calling to things more physical I also grew in size. By the age of 13 I weighed in at over 14 stone. I had spots and eczema – there was no stopping my descent into misery. It was 1967 and I had started to take a real interest in clothes. Unfortunately, this was the era of the mini, and I would look longingly at girls wearing the latest fashions, promising myself that I too would be able to wear such outfits one day. One day never came.

It was at this point that my dieting got out of hand. Although my mother had been enraged at the school doctor for her comments she also had a somewhat ambivalent attitude towards food and weight. One month my mother and I would eat what we wanted and the next our lives would be permeated with diets of all kinds. My father, who never weighed more than seven and a half stone regardless of how much he ate, would also reinforce my mother's ambivalence. He would make negative, hurtful comments about our weight and the way we looked and then, probably because he felt guilty, would bring home two or three family-sized chocolate bars for our rapid consumption. This rather erratic attitude towards food meant my mother and I were constantly either thinking about, on or just finishing a diet. But any external criticism, whether real or simply perceived, was always met with the 'large is healthy' party line.

I was first put on a diet at the age of six. It was a liquid diet comprising a pint of milk, one egg and the juice of an orange. Water, black tea and coffee were generously allowed. We lost weight for our holidays but needless to say gained even more during the holiday itself. By 13 I had tried numerous diets, including the egg, the grapefruit and the rice diet. And of course, let's not forget fasting. This was an era when starvation was a good way to lose weight and crash dieting was seen as a virtue.

My interest in clothes, make-up and boys seemed to be thwarted at every turn. There were simply no fashionable clothes for larger sizes. All I could find were hideous Crimplene outfits. Make-up was impossible because of my skin condition and no self-respecting boy wanted to take any interest in me. My romantic urges were forced into intense and powerful crushes on teachers and actors. I had always wanted to be an actress and I soon realised that if I were to move beyond the chorus I had to develop myself as a character actress, and so my impersonations of Hattie Jacques began, she being the only role model available for a size 16 plus. It doesn't take much imagination to realise that my teens were spent weeping into my pillow, dreaming of being thin, dieting, bingeing and more dieting. As my friends 'snogged' away quite happily at the school disco I would take centre stage with my dancing and joke telling, pretending all was well, only to return home at the end of the evening to cry myself to sleep.

Fourteen, 15 and 16 saw no improvement, although I did manage to use the remains of the hippie era to my advantage by wearing extremely bright caftans with copious amounts of jewellery. Sixteen saw the loss of my virginity. Sadly, this took place not because I was in a loving relationship but because I was so grateful to be looked at by anyone. It was an un-memorable experience which was to be repeated many times over the years in my quest for love, affection and acceptance. I had developed the unhelpful habit of weighing myself daily and my moods and self-esteem rose and fell in line with the needle on the scale. A pound on triggered the spiral of self-loathing and a pound off fed the fantasy of a slim and glorious life. By 17 I had left school as an academic failure.

I spent the following two years pursuing my theatrical

dream and feeding myself a range of prescribed amphetamines in a bid for slimness. It was a time of auditions, roles in fringe companies, touring and sleeping in traditionally awful 'digs' while waiting for my big break. I believed all my problems would vanish automatically once I had shed my weight.

For many people in the performing arts work is inter-mittent, so I worked in shops, wine bars, offices – anywhere I could make some money to tide me over. There were relationships but none which boosted my self-esteem or lasted any length of time. Painfully I came to realise that stardom was not around the next corner and at 20 decided it was time to leave my dreams behind. Perhaps ambition had outstripped talent. Being the eternal optimist I threw myself into a range of jobs. I was an audio secretary, ran an employment agency, got involved in public relations and co-ordinated a fleet of company cars. I also spent much of my time looking for something to wear. Thankfully, the midi was in, which meant I could hide my legs, but finding boots large enough to cover my calves was another matter.

After a series of relationship difficulties I developed what the doctor called 'a nervous stomach'. I was unable to eat anything without feeling sick and my stomach felt as if it were permanently bloated with something resembling a football inside. After ten weeks (and a barium meal to check for ulcers) I was three stone lighter. Suddenly, there was light at the end of the tunnel: I could lose weight. When I was able to eat again I learned to survive on coffee, the odd apple and three packets of cigarettes a day. The pay-off as I saw it came in the guise of a size 10 top and a size 12 bottom. I had made it!

There was no stopping me. I bought trousers, jeans, clingy tops, skirts, dresses, fitted coats, knee-high boots. An Aladdin's Cave opened up and I rushed in to gorge myself on as much as (and in some cases more than) my bank balance could take. Now it was not food which preoccupied me but clothes. Markets, shops and mail order fascinated me as I experimented with shape, colour and style.

My twenty-first year seemed to be full of so much promise. I met and married Peter McMahon, a good-looking Australian, and thought my life was complete. I was flattered that someone as handsome as he would want to go out with me. He turned heads and the slimline me basked in reflected glory. Two years later the marriage was over, but I was still slim.

I now had clothes, bags and shoes stacked from ceiling to floor, in cupboards and under beds. No available space was spared. It never occurred to me to look beyond the clothes. The fact that I was heading towards bulimic behaviour never registered; all that did was the idol of slimness. I found that as long as I stuck to a routine I could control my weight. My routine was to eat as little as possible from Monday to Friday and then to eat as much as I could on Saturday and Sunday. My weight could be maintained as long as nothing altered my routine. Holidays were frightening as it was possible to put on ten pounds in a week. The first day or so would always start out with me desperately trying to eat very little. By the third day with no work to occupy me, I would begin to binge. I would return to work full of panic which would gradually subside as my control returned and the weight came off.

In 1977 I found myself working on reception for Open Door, a youth counselling service in North London. The job came by accident through a friend. It meant meeting the public, being sympathetic to callers, making appointments for people to see a counsellor and doing general administrative work. From the moment I arrived I loved my job. I had found my vocation. I worked hard and soon the director of the service was asking me whether I had ever thought of becoming a counsellor.

I jumped at the chance. I had always been an unofficial agony aunt to everyone. I knew so this was an opportunity to get paid for doing something I loved. I was seconded to a three-year diploma course and my counselling career began. For the next three years I lived and breathed counselling. I went into personal therapy and began looking at my past. The alcoholic father and the highly controlling mother, my experiences of racism, childhood stress, poor academic achievement, low self-esteem and sense of failure all poured out. With each confused and painful memory or disclosure I moved one step nearer to being the kind of person I always wanted to be. I wanted the shy, anxious, easily frightened person inside to match the flamboyant, confident person I presented to the world. There was so much work to do in putting the past to rest and learning how to function in the present that somehow my current eating patterns never seemed to get discussed. I believed there was nothing wrong with my eating – after all, I was slim.

Another turning point came in 1982 when I met Michael, my current partner. We met, as many couples do, through work. I started to put on weight. I couldn't sustain the self-deprivation any longer and Michael liked his food. During the next five years my weight fluctuated dramatically and Michael loved me whatever my shape. I would put on a stone, even two, then panic. Having read Geoffrey Cannon's book *Why Dieting Makes You Fat*, which advocates exercise and a complex carbohydrate diet usually in the form of brown rice and pasta, I started running. At one time I was able to run ten miles and trained four times a week. However, my knees paid a price and I developed cartilage problems. My wardrobe was now full of clothes of differing sizes and I still weighed myself daily.

In 1985 we moved to Blackheath and the current phase of my life began. I became Director of Public Relations for Turning Point, a national substance misuse and mental health charity. My career was going from success to success. I loved what I was doing and in 1987 I was asked to become Associate Director (Therapeutic Resources) for a private sector provider.

By now my weight was back up to 13 stone and I was a size 18. All my other clothes were packed away waiting for the day I would become slim again.

I had kept my counselling going by seeing a few clients on

a voluntary basis and, in 1988, I decided it was time to become self-employed. So I started my business on the first of October 1988. My practice thrived. I was good at what I did and people passed the word around. I lost a baby through miscarriage and had some brief therapy to help me deal with this. I also decided it was time to give up smoking. I was 34 and was beginning to acknowledge my mortality. Three packs a day was a lot by anyone's standards. So I set myself a date to stop on 9 January the following year. I wanted Christmas and the New Year well and truly over before taking on what I saw as a monumental task. I used my time to focus on the reasons why I smoked, which cigarettes I would miss most and the kinds of coping strategies I could employ when the time came. I signed up for more professional training and January came. I managed to give up smoking and also to put on four stone in the first year. It was now 1989 and I was 17 stone. Shopping was painful as I was back to having little choice, and Evans became my haven. By 1990 my career continued on the up but I felt desperate about my weight. Yet much to my surprise I did not return to smoking; this was one habit I had truly put to rest.

Something had to be done. I sat down one day and realised that I was not applying my therapeutic knowledge to my attitude towards my weight. Out went the scales as I had been ruled by them for too long. With no daily weigh-ins, a sense of relief and also of disorientation and fear came into my life. After all, this ritual had been part of my life for so long. Who was I if I was not defined by what I weighed? I examined my thinking style and realised that if I did not truly accept myself how could I expect others to? I could 'pretend' all was well but true acceptance meant liking myself regardless of what anyone else thought. Although bullied as a child I had never experienced the kind of public taunts that so many large people suffer with. When I thought about this I wondered whether presenting myself in such a confident manner had been my defence. I may have felt awful but I never behaved like a victim and was therefore never treated like one. Perhaps my 'pretence' had brought some benefits.

So I used self-acceptance techniques such as consciously telling myself that I am a fallible human being, that I like myself regardless of how other people see me. I reminded myself that if other people had a problem with my weight it was their problem not mine. It only became a problem if I chose to give the control for my life and my happiness to others. I tried to pick up on all the 'shoulds', 'musts' and 'have tos' that I was limiting myself and my life by. For example, thoughts such as 'I must always be approved of by others.' This meant keeping a daily log of those times I felt negative about myself and asking myself what thoughts were going through my mind at the time and then challenging those that were self-defeating in origin. Affirmations came thick and plentiful. The good days got longer and the bad days got shorter; gradually my feelings inside began to match the person I showed to the world.

My career developed apace. I became a British Association for Counselling Accredited Counsellor and Counselling Supervisor and more recently a Fellow. I also became a British Association for Behavioural and Cognitive Psychotherapies Accredited Cognitive-Behavioural Psychotherapist. Each year saw additional qualifications added to my CV. I even signed up for an Open University Psychology Degree. If ever there was a case of 'physician, heal thyself', this was it.

For two years I had been writing for local magazines and I now expanded my writing. I became News Editor for a major professional journal and soon resuscitated my media work. I became a regular on Anglia Television's *The Time, The Place*; provided interviews on a range of subjects for publications as diverse as the *Sun* and *The Times*, *Woman's Own* and *Marie-Claire*; took part in regular radio programmes and wrote my first book. I also discovered that things were beginning to change on the clothes front. Shops such as Ann Harvey and Elvi were added to my shopping haunts, Evans revamped its image and mail order began for larger sizes.

One day, having weighed myself for the first time in many months at a friend's house, I found that two more stone had crept on. Although I weighed 19 stone I realised I had become the person I wanted to be. My career could not have been more successful. I was now Agony Aunt for *YES!* magazine, had a regular weekly slot on Channel 5's *Espresso* and was writing and editing books and articles for a range of publications. What's more, I no longer worried about what the scales said. I still needed to challenge my negative thinking as years of putting myself down could not be wiped out quite so easily. Therapy is hard work, and changing thinking styles means a commitment.

Finding Ken Smith Designs also helped: a wonderful shop in the centre of London which stocks a range of clothing from all over the world specially for larger sizes. At last there is a designer shop for large women. I no longer have smaller size clothes anywhere in the house and my local charity shop has benefited from my massive de-cluttering exercise. To keep such clothes would mean I was not living in the present as I would still be believing that I'm not good enough just the way I am. Self-acceptance really is the key to success.

I have a wonderful partner, good friends and a job I love with as much variety as my Geminian nature can stand. I really like myself and with each day I realise that success comes from within. If I want something I set goals, make plans and go for it. There are more books to write, more people to meet and definitely more clothes to buy.

Being Fat

Miriam Margolyes

I've been fat all my life and I expect to die fat. But I'm not fat inside. I'm a little darting thing with quick movements to match my quick mind and when I realised I was fat, which was probably when I was eleven, I decided to use it to my advantage.

My mother was fat and my father slender and trim. He was also tone deaf and I have inherited his dark eyes and his inability to hold a tune. But because, as Oscar Wilde said, it is all women's tragedy that they grow to resemble their mother, it is inevitable that my pendulous breasts (size 44E), sagging belly and multiple chins have been a feature of my silhouette.

Do I mind? Of course I mind, very much. It is neither socially, sexually nor psychologically acceptable to be fat; it can also be medically unsafe and actuarially challenged – it raises your insurance premiums! So the fat person is obliged to make an adjustment of some kind, either to be continually guilty or continually dieting. If you're Jewish (as I am) you manage both. You also make a joke of it, quickly interposing a self-denigrating remark before anyone else can puncture the self-esteem which lies encased in blubber. But of course there is another truth, the truth about feeling sexy, desired, energetic and amusing. I feel all those things too.

Once I was helping a blind man at a railway station and as I took his arm I explained that I too was handicapped: 'I'm fat,' I said. Many years later, when I toured India with *Dickens' Women*, a blind man came backstage to meet me. He told me how much he enjoyed my vocal range and the variety of my characterisations. 'But I'm fat, you know,' I said, 'let me give you a tour of my body', and I took his hands and allowed them to feel my bulk from top to bottom. 'My goodness,' he exclaimed, 'you are fat.' I acknowledged that I was and felt a little surprised that my voice didn't show it.

Fatness is not a state of mind and mustn't be allowed to become so. It is a state of body and society has decided that it's a reprehensible state of body. I remember my father saying that he would not be surprised if, in the future, doctors refused to treat fat people since he believed their illnesses were often caused by their own wilful actions. He was a doctor of the old school who did not smoke or drink, ate in moderation and survived until he was 96. I am quite sure that I will not live so long and it is my bulk which will kill me. So why do I remain fat?

People ask me sometimes if I remain fat to preserve my place in show business, as if my weight were the only repository of my talent. I would be much the same sort of actress, I think, if I were half my size, but it is certainly true that I might find it harder to get work. There are millions of brilliant, thin actresses – not so many of the larger variety. (It's not that I think I'm brilliant – I am!)

Do I make this kind of absurdly conceited statement because I am covering up for inner insecurity? I don't know, but speculation is pointless. Any actress who works is damn lucky; I would certainly be prepared to be out of work if I could be thin – so far it hasn't happened.

Everyone is typecast, of course – no use railing against Fate for making me fat and talented, instead of just talented. I'll never play Juliet, but I played the Nurse and I hope I will again. You *never* get to be the love interest if you're fat – but as long as I do *in life*, I can cope. Bitterness makes you ugly – and I won't be fat *and* ugly.

Fat people are the butt of jokes, are scorned and laughed at. Yet I have always found that my human contacts were warm and full of laughter. Not cruel but loving. My nature is a sunny one, my life is surrounded with kindness and comfort and a considerable amount of joy. Therefore, I would say that I have not allowed my weight to come between me and the wider world. My fat isn't an obsession, it is a regret.

When I see a fat woman in the street I think to myself, 'That's my part.' I feel a certain fellowship with her, a knowledge that her thighs are rubbing against each other painfully in the summer, that she feels obliged to change her knickers every day (naturally), that she has to take particular care of personal freshness; that she looks to see her back view in case the roll of fat under her bra distorts the line of her jumper. I know that she will try to eat a little bit secretly so that rude strangers won't call out 'You shouldn't be eating that' as the last Kit Kat folds into her mouth. I also know that the Fat Woman is probably more compassionate and quicker to laughter than her thin sister, that she will have fewer lines on her face and a fresher complexion, with skin that is smoother to the touch. So, at the end of it all let us try to see through each other, be philosophical about the things we can't change, take care of our health as best we can and when making love, don't squash our partners.

The Great Weight Debate

Betty Woods

Let me paint a picture of myself. I am a 23-year-old artist, involved with SIZE, co-editing and designing the magazine *Freesize*, while freelancing with a textiles studio designing children's wear. Born in Wales, I moved to Winchester in 1993 to study at Winchester School of Art.

From an early age I knew I was artistic. I knew that there was something in painting, drawing – whatever – that attracted me. It is something that can never leave you, because it is you. It's in your system. There was no dispute as to which direction I would take throughout school. Art was the 'favourite' – from GCSE through to 'A' level. Then I went on to Carmarthenshire College of Technology and Art, completing a one-year foundation diploma course. That is where I really came into myself. It was where my fascination with the body began, as life drawing was a definite fixture within the course. After that I was lucky enough to be accepted at Winchester School of Art where I studied a fine art printmaking degree, specialising in photographic screenprint, digital media, photographic and mixed media.

This was where the fine line between my work and my views about the body fused to become one quest. This was where I accepted my weight 'problem' and just got on with it. My work became a vehicle for my questions around the 'great weight debate'. All the negative experiences that I had previously endured because I was fat were now my subjects for dissection. My work became a kind of therapy where I could work through anxieties, and I felt this could benefit not only myself but also the viewer. This in turn became a vehicle for challenging the viewer, trying to provoke a response. It gave me the chance to ask all the questions I'd left unexamined all this time; inspecting all the insults that society has had the 'right' to bestow on me, asking, why have I let society dump their body hatred onto my lap?

Fat issues are very close to my heart, but this is something I find hard to explain. It is as if through all the negative experiences I have encountered something very strong yet fragile has been created; something that can bring a lump to my throat, and a tear to my cheek. My fat is as much an emotional thing as it is physical. There is something about being fat, feeling fat, knowing that I am fat which creates this very precious feeling. I am just so proud that at the age of 23 I actually believe in myself, that I love 'me' as the whole package. I have bonded with myself. Sometimes I could cry when I get these feelings, but it is because they are so very, very important to me. When I look back on all the years I was bullied, tormented and segregated for being fat, it makes me proud that I didn't let 'them' win. It gives me great pleasure in announcing to Brett, Oliver and all the other narrow-minded boys (at school), that though they thought their torments would eventually break me, all they have done is make me one hell of a strong, secure, well-balanced, considerate and triumphant woman. I have reclaimed my 'title' from them all, turning it from a negative to a descriptive term – FAT. My fat is something that has slowly and gently surrounded my being, which has grown with me, grown into me; it is involved in so much I do, so much I speak of – and all that I am. I have had to fight for acceptance, which in turn has made me an assertive, confident and mentally alert individual.

The titles of my works are very important to me. They bring the piece together, informing the viewer of my intentions, and interpreting how very angry and sometimes aggressive my beliefs can be. Titles such as *Lard Arse, Can You Pinch More Than an Inch, Fatbird, Sniff Yourself Slim* and *Donuts* create a provocative tone. I am not *encouraging* these negative words to be used as they were intended; but rather than using venomous language against the perpetrators, I am using *their* language to shock and retaliate.

My *Donuts* piece originated through a heated debate with a work colleague. He repeatedly insinuated that 'fat birds' were fat due to an over indulgence in doughnuts. Obviously, my colleague was 'only having a laugh', but such a remark goes far deeper than this, implying that anyone fat is nothing more than a glutton who is 'out of control' and takes up too much space. I wanted to change this negative portrayal of 'eating is greedy', to a positive, blissful and pleasurable experience. Hence *Donuts* – a piece of work celebrating the simple enjoyment of food. I wanted to express that there is no need to feel guilty for eating. I wanted the model to be as scrumptious as the doughnut itself: gorgeous, triumphant and jubilant. Why should we be insulted by other people's hang-ups? I believe that we can make a difference within society by embracing the power of self-acceptance, and reclaiming our freedom of choice.

Another piece of work I have exhibited is an image from the Wonderbra advertisement featuring the supermodel Eva with the slogans 'Hello Boys', 'Mind if I bring a couple of friends', and 'It's Okay, they're with me'. I decided to replace the ideal with the real – and changed Eva for myself. I wanted to challenge the viewer, to ask what it really meant to have this advertising ideal replaced. The piece had a strong political context, yet it was tongue-in-cheek. I like that about my work – that there is this underlying tone of humour, creating a shared understanding, which encourages the viewer into questioning their own beliefs and judgements. I want my work to be occupied by an intelligence that makes them ashamed of their responses, and dismayed by their shame.

My work is mainly photographic enhanced digital media. It centres around nudes in a bid to alter perceptions, which in a way is an act of defiance but not self-loathing. I never quite know where the boundaries lie in relation to how much of the artist the viewer should see, yet I have such emotional ties that sometimes I worry that I am not giving the viewer enough space to decide for themselves. I don't think that I can work any other way. There is an element of standing up naked in front of the crowd, standing up and letting myself be counted – 'confronting' the 'confronter'.

Fat is simply a descriptive word. Just like tall, short, thin, black, white, lesbian, gay, heterosexual, it describes an element of what we are. I am sick and tired of one element being placed above another. I'm tired of one ideal being raised by stamping on another. The term fat is no different in the 'better or worse' categories. I'm not saying that fat is better than anything else, but it can definitely be as fabulous, gorgeous, stunning and everything else that the term 'slim' stands for. My work aims to break down the barriers of fattism and help others like myself find the confidence to stand up for what they believe is right. By emphasising the positive picture, I hope that it will cause them to rethink their attitudes and end the persecution of anyone who cannot or does not wish to conform to the 'ideal'. Unlike society, I appreciate myself. I am empowered by my body with its ample, boundless flesh and succulent proportions. I can look at myself through unbiased eyes, without prejudice, scorn, insult or rejection. Unfortunately, through lack of education, ignorance or intense rudeness, there are people who do look at my body with such thoughts – but why should I allow such prejudices to harm me? Beauty is in the eye of the beholder – a fact which unfortunately many have yet to realise.

I do not stake any claims, nor do I have any overblown expectations about changing the world. By asking questions, I hope to alert others to these pressing issues. By demonstrating vigilance, scepticism and the refusal to be fobbed off, I hope to offer an example of intelligent enquiry; of how to stand up and be counted, and of refusing to let individuality die.

The Devil and the Deep Blue Sea

Shelley Bovey

I am afraid of being thin. I was, once, very thin indeed. I suppose I would have been about seven or eight, and I couldn't be bothered to eat because I had better things to do. A small, black and white photograph shows me with my father and my little brother, a picture taken on an obviously hot day, with me, all skinny arms and legs, grinning and holding in my arms a huge ginger and white cat. (I know I said the photo was black and white, but you can tell.) It brings forward memories of that careless, carefree part of childhood when I roamed, unfettered and unafraid, through the woods and fields of the countryside It was a pastoral idyll, a lost time. I recall wading in streams and plunging into their clear waters clad in shorts and T-shirts, longing to learn to swim but they were too shallow. I rode cows – legged up onto their bony backs by other children who thought I was mad – but I yearned for ponies and this was the nearest I could get. Cow-riding was a dangerous pastime but who cared?

There was so much for a country child to do that going home for meals was a bore. I was anorexic in the literal sense: I had no appetite, no desire for food and I may even have been a little malnourished, though not seriously. If it happened today I would probably be a patient at some paediatric eating disorders clinic. Caring professionals would look into the pressures in my life; the media would be blamed for portraying such unreasonable images of ideal femininity that even eight-year-olds fell victim to anorexia. As it was, a thin child in the fifties had no aesthetic body-consciousness. I read recently that girl children become aware of their bodily imperfections as early as three years old. All I can say is that it didn't happen then and if it's happening now, then what are their parents exposing them to?

My mother was anxious about my lack of appetite and tried to tempt me with lovingly prepared food which served only as an irritant. I couldn't wait to get down from the table and be outside again. I was weighed and charted and given Radio Malt (thick, sweet, dark brown sticky stuff, eaten off a spoon) to build me up but no great fuss was made. And then suddenly I was 11 and I had become plump. I was rather astonished really. I hadn't actually noticed it happening. I could still run and jump, climb high trees and ride, though I had progressed from cows to ponies (other people's which I rode illicitly in the chilly, breaking dawn, bareback and with a halter I'd saved my pocket money to buy).

This 'puppy fat' didn't bother me at primary school. As long as our handwriting was neat and our hair was brushed, we cared nothing for appearances. We were too preoccupied with our storybook adventures in the great rolling folds and woods of Burnham Beeches where the school stood, tiny and alone. But after the eleven plus I had to go into town each day to the grammar school, a long bus ride away. And I learned there, for the first time, that being fat was a Bad Thing. Did it make a difference, I wonder, that cultural switch from country to town? Were the pre-teen town girls of the late fifties already more aware than I knew how to be? Certainly they stood for hours in front of the cloakroom mirrors backcombing their bouffants. They pulled their school skirts in with wide tight belts which the teachers made them remove. I suppose they were conscious of their figures. I suppose it was important to them. Childhood was beginning, even then, to change.

Being different is the worst kind of trial for a child. I already wore round, pink, wire-rimmed National Health glasses and was none too happy about those. But I'd had them since I was four and largely grown accustomed to them. This fatness, though, was different and I discovered on the first day at my new school that it was something to be ashamed of. The games mistress, measuring us for our uniform aertex gym-shirts, called out that I was a 'big girl'. Humiliation shot through me like a hot flush. It was the first sign of years of victimisation. I know now that some fat adults cannot endure fat children; rather than empathise they are repelled by them. This teacher was one such person. After that I learned to live with the constant feeling that I had committed a fairly grave sin.

Messages received at that age burn their way into the mind, like the brand mark in a cow's ear. I remember turning miserably to the girl next to me in line – an earnest, stolid sort of person who looked as though she might offer comfort. 'I'm fat,' I said, 'and nobody else is.' She looked at me with consternation, totally unable to deny the truth of my bald statement. 'Well,' she said consolingly, 'you've got nice feet.' To this day I have great confidence in my feet. I will flaunt them at anyone.

Strangely enough I don't remember being called names like Fatso or Four Eyes at school – maybe they have been edited out by a selective memory trying to mitigate the pain. Because pain there was, from that first day, and humiliation and ignominy and the knowledge that whatever I did, I could not be like the others. The teachers, especially the evil games mistress, created a kind of self-fulfilling prophecy for me. Though I didn't feel I had any problem with physical education (I am still as supple as an octopus), clearly *they* felt I did. 'Running and jumping are difficult for Shelley', says an old school report. 'But she might, with practice, throw the discus.'

That running and jumping were difficult was news to me but I was saved from being typecast as a hefty discus thrower by my first attempt. I chucked the thing with vigour in the wrong direction; it cracked the shin bone of one of my class mates and sent her writhing in agony to the ground. The answer to their problem (for it certainly wasn't mine) was to put me on a diet. I had to report regularly to the school matron who was more fearful than any childhood bogeyman. She had a whip-thin waist, the features of a maddened hawk and the compassion of an executioner. And she was the first of a long line of medics to predict the most dire health problems.

Every woman who has dieted, especially from puberty, knows what it is like. The extremes of hunger, the emptiness that is never filled, the coldness, the loneliness. Those latter feelings may seem unrelated to dieting but they are an inextricable part of it, physical and psychological. I was unhappy and introverted though the face I presented to the world was that of the jolly clown who was always good for a prank or a merry jape to make others laugh. This façade got me into trouble but made me popular, giving my classmates the exquisite *schadenfreude* of watching me being given detention yet again. And of course the dieting made me shrink, then swell again in a repetitive, rhythmical pattern. But I knew I had to try to become thin. The message had permeated every layer of my conscious and unconscious mind. After all, I'd never get anywhere in life if I was fat. Everyone said so.

At that stage there was still a definite split between my own perception of my body and that of others. I liked it. It worked for me, it did what I wanted – Okay, so I couldn't buy fashionable clothes but I wasn't particularly interested in fashionable clothes. I never looked at myself and saw hideous rolls of fat. I just saw – well, me. Other people defined me by my size but I did not. The problem wasn't my body; it was the fact that people set me apart because of it. This, of course, is the root of every fat person's pain but I didn't know that then. It would never have occurred to me as a child that the very fat teacher who made an example of me in front of my class may have been feeling immensely hurt herself. I didn't even *want* to be thin; I just thought I *needed* to be in order to placate and please the rest of the world.

What amazes and angers me now is that when I look back at school photographs I see that I was not even fat. Not really, properly fat. I was about size 16–18 which meant I did not stand out hugely from my peers. But I believed and internalised the disapproval of the masses and it did its corrosive work. I think they were even surprised when I got into university. Or did I imagine they were? Being fat can bring its own particular paranoia, but just because you're paranoid it doesn't mean they're not out to get you.

I didn't have boyfriends. I assumed that fat girls did not and another self-fulfilling prophecy was born. My teenage years were spent at home alone, listening to Radio Luxembourg and wondering what it must be like to look like Marianne Faithfull. But then I met a man who did not think my size had anything to do with who I was or with what was real and essential. We fell in love and together we faced the world. I was pretty heavy by then and the pressure was on (though not from my beloved), to lose weight for my wedding. And by this time I wanted to, I really wanted to be – not thin, that wouldn't seem right, but thinner. Egged on by my future mother-in-law I went to the doctor who put me on a 1000 calorie a day diet and weighed me weekly. It was so easy. I lost four stone in a year and weighed ten and a half stone on my wedding day. Curiously, and out of step with the medical mythology that still prevails, this doctor did not think I should try to get to my 'ideal' weight (about seven and a half stone, I think it is). 'Don't go below ten stone,' he commanded. And I never did. But ten and a half was very nice and I could buy my going away outfit from C&A like everyone else.

So how come two years later I weighed 15 stone? Actually it was 15 stone $3^{1}/_{2}$ lbs and the figure is graven on my brain because when it was written down (on my antenatal card at my first ever check-up, six weeks pregnant), my horror, disgust and disbelief were such that I started dieting immediately. I think this was the point of the shift: from being unhappy only because of the persecution, to beginning to hate my body for what it was. The judgement of others obliterated my core feelings that I was all right as I was, their opinion overshadowed my own convictions and I entered a new state of helplessness. I lost three stone in that pregnancy and after it I put that card in the medicine cabinet where it sat, silent witness to the unthinkable. For I knew that never again – and what a wonderful relief to know salvation – never again would I reach that terrible, obscene weight. And I had my next child and maintained the weight, even lost some more, so that I was about 13 stone just before she was born. Huge baby with all her baggage and me only weighing 13 stone. You see, I told myself, it can be done.

With an inevitability that was to become heart-sinkingly familiar, I grew fatter again and started my third pregnancy at 16 stone. Horror upon horror from the medics. 'You shouldn't be pregnant,' they said. 'It's a terrible risk being pregnant at that weight.' (Subtext: best you have an abortion.) That, I think, was the nadir: that denial of my child and of my body's ability to bring him safely into the world. They were so wrong, too. I had normal deliveries, no drugs, no stitches, and breast-fed for years. My body worked for, not against me and I was comfortable with all the physical intimacies of childbirth, but after the last child was weaned I began to hate my fatness and struggled helplessly against it.

In the eighties I went back to my work in journalism. Things had changed. The fattism which had sprung up in the sixties had put down deep roots. I worked as a reporter for Radio 4 and loved it, but one day the controller's secretary came into my office, shut the door and told me that I should know that it was being said, high up where it mattered, that I must lose weight because I didn't 'present a good image of the BBC'. Bugger that, I thought, and went back to print journalism, contributing to newspapers and magazines, working from home, where I couldn't be seen. Except that my contract with one magazine required me to attend monthly editorial meetings and lunches in smart restaurants where twig-thin editors pretended to eat and bitched about other women's weight. They even wanted to do a make-over on me for the mag – a before and after diet piece. Ha! I'd had enough. Turning point had arrived.

I wrote a letter to the deputy editor, a woman I liked enormously. In it I ranted about the raw deal given to fat women: the prejudice, the discrimination, the pain, the damage done to lives. It was really just to get it off my chest, but she rang me. 'Write about it,' she said, and bemused, I set to it. It was breaking new ground for a women's magazine and it appeared, uncut, full of rage and entitled 'Being Fat Is Not a Sin – a Plea for An End to Prejudice'. Letters poured in and a publisher asked me to write a book about it

The book (called *Being Fat Is Not a Sin*, after the article) was the first of its kind in Britain and attracted a lot of publicity. I found myself giving a great many media interviews. I was frequently surprised by the tone of them which tended to begin like this: 'Well, Shelley, you're obviously fat and happy/proud to be fat/happy to be the size you are.' Where had they got that idea from? The book had been a battle cry on behalf of fat women everywhere, demanding equal rights and equal respect for them, truly a plea for an end to prejudice. It described the pain of being ostracised, marginalised and condemned. It said Stop and Enough and Judge Not. Nowhere did I say I was happy to be fat.

But at that point I didn't know myself very well. I knew I didn't want to be thin. After all, my adult identity is tied up in being a big woman. People see me as an Earth Mother and I like that. They come and drink tea in my kitchen and weep upon my shoulder when they need to and I'm glad to have a broad shoulder to provide for them. And of all the roles in my life motherhood is the most important. Being a mother to my children and being an Earth Mother became intertwined and I do not think I could fulfil those roles in my own particular way if I were thin. Self-image is, I believe, more important than what other people dictate, and though most women claim they would love to be slim, I know it wouldn't suit me. Oh yes, I know that people would admire and flatter and feel that at last I had joined the human race as society designed it to be. But *I* would not feel right. I would feel somehow insubstantial if I were thin. I would feel conformist and invisible and indistinguishable from all the other thin, obedient women who guard their weight and daily step on the scales. So I fear thinness.

And so I agreed with the interviewers – that yes, I was happy being fat. And when asked, as I often was, if I would take a magic pill to make me thin overnight, I said no, and gave carefully considered reasons for my answer. I remember being on one television programme with Jo Brand, who, when we were asked that particular question, said laconically: 'I'd rather have a cake'! And at the time, after I'd given my right-on philosophical response, I couldn't help feeling uncomfortably that there was somehow more honesty in hers. I did not consider at that point what my answer would have been had I been asked if I would take a pill to make me *less fat*. Ah, there's the rub.

Meanwhile the repercussions from the book gathered their own momentum. I was asked to bring out another, bigger edition and more interviews and articles followed. Inevitably I was challenged by those who took the mainstream view that Fat Is Bad, but also by a tiny section of the now burgeoning size acceptance movement. Some felt I had sold out by retitling the new edition of my book *The Forbidden Body: Why Being Fat Is Not a Sin*. There were reasons for this: I had received a number of letters from readers who found it difficult to ask for it in bookshops. Many women have a problem with the word fat, for it is resonant with negative connotations and painful memories. Besides, I admit that I have not yet come to the point of owning it myself. I use it intermittently, interspersed with 'big' and 'large', and though I have been slated for my ambivalence, I stand by my need to be honest.

And so, through my work, I came to realise that there are many shades of grey between the black and white certainties of fat hatred and fat pride. What is often not recognised is that some of us – and I know now that I am one – would like to be less fat than we are. This is not a betrayal: we can sympathise with those who feel too small at 4'11" or find being 6' an awkward height for a woman. We ourselves might consider such women delightfully petite or enviably tall; nevertheless we respect that *they* are not comfortable being so far outside the norm. And it is not easy to be *very* fat, to be such a long way outside the boundaries of social, medical and aesthetic acceptability. I had thought that not wanting to be thin, yet not wanting to be as large as I am put me somewhere between the Devil and the deep blue sea. I had thought it put me outside both camps and once I identified my feelings about my size, I did not dare share them. If I told those of average weight that I would like to be less fat, then no doubt they would have had a plethora of dietary remedies. On the other hand, I thought that if I confessed to my colleagues in the size acceptance movement that I was not entirely comfortable with my bulk, then they might ostracise me.

In fact, understanding my true position has been a source of enormous liberation. I have broken the bonds of two different but equally confining ideals. I want to deal in reality. There comes a point for many women when they feel what I can only describe as a sense of growing out of their skin. This can be physiological or psychological and it can happen at vastly differing sizes. There are plenty of women who don't feel like that at 25 stone and they move freely and fluidly, they dance, they run, they are not restricted. On the other hand, some women feel they have outgrown their skin at 16 or 17 stone. But for me it came when I could no longer do cartwheels. As long as I could do cartwheels, I couldn't be too fat, could I?

Paradoxically, being free to be honest, to say 'Actually, I'm not wildly ecstatic being this fat but there's little I can do about it because diets don't work,' has been the key to freedom. I have more true acceptance of myself than when I was glibly agreeing that I was happy to be fat and wondering why such confident sounding words didn't *feel* right deep inside. I have learned to live in my body rather than to exist in it, to dwell in it with my mind and soul and not to strain against it as though it were some kind of incarceration.

So I am not celebrating being fat any more than I would celebrate being thin. Being fat is not what defines me; what I have achieved and who I have become are what define me. I have had everything I've wanted out of life; all those things that I was told years ago were out of the reach of the fat girl. I have a long and happy marriage, the children I longed for, wonderful friends and a successful career.

And I am celebrating the gifts that have come directly from being fat: riches I would not have had if I had not endured the pain and isolation of cultural ostracism. I'm celebrating all the other fat women with whom I have such a close bond; all the precious friendships and connections that have come about through the work I have done. I'm celebrating my success in a world that hates fat; the strength I've gained through learning to stand up to my detractors; the fact that when people tell me that I have a weight problem I can say 'I don't have a problem, you do. Deal with it.'

Perhaps somewhat to my surprise, I'm celebrating being me!

Nobody's Fall-Guy
Identifying and Resisting Anti-fat Prejudices within Western Culture

Angela Kennedy

Every age can be said to develop its own peculiar forms of pathology, which are expressed – sometimes in very exaggerated forms – within the cultures of that age. For example, when we see the depiction of nude women in European oil paintings from the sixteenth and seventeenth centuries, they are often very fleshy – not because most women of the time were necessarily fat, but because there was a cultural preference for fat women. Their corpulence is likely to have indicated the wealth of the commissioner of the painting (rather like the plump farm animals often depicted in oils), as well as the sexual desire of the male viewers of such paintings, a forerunner to present day erotica.

Even late nineteenth- and early twentieth-century, pornographic photographs were of bigger women, with expansive, cellulite-covered thighs that today would be vigorously scrubbed with strange rubber contraptions. I am not arguing that the sexual objectification of women in such images, whether they be fat or thin, is right or desirable. I am using these comparisons only to place the current obsession with thinness within its cultural and historical context.

Attitudes change, and today, when discrimination and prejudice on grounds of race and disability are now illegal and denounced, it appears that fat-hatred is the last safe prejudice of so-called liberal societies.

But why on earth should fat bodies engender such disapproval? I do not, yet, and may never profess to have the definite answer to such a question. However, the answer may be found by examining why thin bodies have become such objects of desire.

Some feminists link the prevalence of anorexia nervosa with the 'dualistic' notions inherited from philosophers such as Plato, Aristotle and Descartes, in which the body is seen merely as a brute envelope to the mind, something that must be controlled. Whereas the anorexic does indeed exert amazing control over her body, denying it essential nourishment in order to make it thin, the fat person can actually be seen as subversive, actively resisting such cultural compulsions, refusing to behave in the ways expected of us. And subversive people are often hated: for being 'different', and because their actions appear to rebuke those who buy in – consciously or unconsciously – to societal obsessions.

There is also a gender dimension to hatred of fat. Some psychoanalysts have linked 'fear' of fatness to repressed memories of an infantile erotic dependence on the mother's body, terrifying to the now adult mind. But a specifically feminist understanding of the fixation with thinness relates to the social pressure on women to take up less space: a taboo against women having 'too much' of physical or metaphysical space or resources that, in a patriarchy, men believe belong to them.

This has particular resonance for me because I am what is often considered a 'fat' woman. I have suffered from a form of hypothyroidism since the age of 16. Definitions of 'fat' are very complex and unstable but for women, dress sizes are often used as an indicator of 'obesity'. I am usually a size 20, but even the physical dimensions of dress sizes themselves are culturally and historically specific, and particularly subject to complexity and instability. Basically, like many – possibly most – women, I have, as part of my wardrobe, a size 16 T-shirt and an old, curry-stained size 30 towelling dressing gown, and they both fit me the same.

With a background in the study of gender, I am undertaking a research degree with a view to obtaining a PhD, but

I also hope my work will serve to validate the experiences of fat women. Very little work seems to have been done by academic feminists about fat women's lives, and certainly very little work by fat women themselves; an enormous gap needs to be filled.

I know from my own experience, and that of many other fat women I know, that at some point we will certainly be called 'Fatty' as we walk past a building site. That is not to say that thinner women do not get harassed in threatening and demoralising ways, only that fat women can predict with some confidence the nature of such encounters. And so, the everyday experiences of fat women often mean that they are waiting to be hailed, identified and designated as fat by others. The aim of my current research is to explore the effects of such attitudes on the lives of fat women: in particular how we are designated as fat, how we feel about this, and the ways in which women resist the very negative connotations about those designations.

Fascination with the thin body has become widespread with the advent of communication technologies. And within twentieth-century Western culture, disapproval does appear to be reserved far more for fat women than fat men. Within North American cinema, for example, male actors such as Nick Nolte, William Hurt or (the lovely) John Travolta, may become thicker in body and still retain romantic leads, while women have to maintain a thin body for these roles. In fact, fatter men are often given all sorts of lead roles in a way that fat women are not – Orson Welles, John Belushi, Marlon Brando, John Goodman, Bob Hoskins, Danny DeVito, Robbie Coltrane...

Fat women, on the other hand, are relegated to supporting roles, there to illustrate a point, not as subjects in their own right – and hardly ever as romantic or desirable leads. There are exceptions, which I'll come to later, but these are few and far between. Far, far more often on the movie screen, the fat woman is conspicuous by her absence. Even if fat women are desired by others in real life (as we are), cultural displeasure projected onto us is so complex and wide-reaching that to feature a fat woman as an object of desire on camera would be dangerously subversive – which is just not the function of Hollywood film.

There are of course many mediums where such anxieties surface. For example in the TV show *Friends*, where Monica (Courtney Cox) gets to be two characters: the present-day extremely thin chef and the greedy fat girl, never present but always referred to unkindly – even by the thin Monica herself – in the past tense. Abhorrence to fatness is manifested in all forms of media: advertisement, comedy, drama, news items, and health promotions campaigns. But I have mentioned Hollywood film specifically, because the research I have undertaken in my previous work relates to this extremely popular and pervasive medium.

Two films that I have studied illustrate very clearly some of the unconscious fears projected onto the bodies of fat women. Interestingly both films, products of the 1990s, allow their protagonists to show some kindness to the fat female characters, but only to show the audience the 'sensitivity' of the protagonists. The female lead in *Heathers* is played by Winona Ryder, and her male co-star is Christian Slater, while *What's Eating Gilbert Grape?* stars Johnny Depp and Juliette Lewis. The beautiful faces and slim bodies of these young actors are in stark contrast to the largeness (and sadly, the contrived ugliness) of the fat women acting in the supporting character roles of both films: Martha and Gilbert Grape's mom.

Heathers could be described as a satire on the cult of the 'American teenager'. Ryder plays a popular girl in high school, who nevertheless is keenly aware of how fragile popularity can be. Her psychotic boyfriend (Slater), with her unwitting help, murders some other popular pupils, framing their deaths as suicides. The dead pupils, however, gain cult status among the others, and it is here that the character of

Martha is used to frame the film's message.

Martha Dunstock is known throughout the film as Martha Dumptruck. Even the film credits include the nickname beside the character's surname (evidently feeling the need to labour the point). Portrayed as unattractive and pathetically grateful for any attention she is given, she unwittingly provides Slater with information enabling him to murder a pupil. Later, when the cult status of the 'suicides' becomes apparent, Martha attempts her own suicide by walking into the path of traffic. But her attempt is shown as a failure. At the end of the film Martha is bruised and disabled, in an electric wheelchair. Ryder's character, having finished her voyage of self-realisation (and killed off Slater), rejects the school Prom night and instead invites Martha to stay in with a video and popcorn. Martha gratefully accepts and the closing scenes show Ryder walking down the corridor while Martha encircles her like a planet around the sun.

The image of Martha in her wheelchair, an object of pity for Ryder and for us, the audience, signifies to us fears of being different, of not being beautiful, of not being loved or respected. Martha is the person we are all frightened of becoming. She is given no means of solving her own predicament by the film-maker. And, though some of us in the audience are fat, or disabled, or both, *we* may fear Martha, and are invited to consider Ryder's protagonist's journey of self-discovery as our own even if, in physical and social reality, we are more like Martha.

In *What's Eating Gilbert Grape?* Johnny Depp is the middle son in a dysfunctional small town North American family. The elder son is at college, the younger son is mentally disabled (two sisters are also present, though merely as additional signs of the 'problem family') and we find out later that the father hanged himself some years before. But Gilbert's greatest resentment is towards his mother. She is very fat, becoming so, we are told, after her husband's death, and has not left the house since. She is so fat that she has (apparently) impaired the foundations of the house and the scene reflecting this is noteworthy, because it is only when Mom stands up and stamps her foot in anger that Depp's character realises the house is unstable. Mom's anger has become physically too much for the house.

The character of Mom functions as a spectacle. Depp allows small boys to come and peep at her watching television. People stare at her when she ventures out of the house on the single occasion when she needs to collect her younger son from the sheriff's office. Yet when Depp becomes romantically involved with Juliette Lewis's character, he initially refuses to let her meet Mom. When they do finally meet Mom is mortified and attempts to explain away her size to Lewis: 'I wasn't always like this.' Lewis, standing with Depp looking down on Mom in her chair, is portrayed as gracious and kind, yet the unconscious positioning of both leading characters, gazing down on Mom throughout the whole exchange, evokes an uneasy realisation that this intercourse is not between three equal human beings. Mom is presented entirely as lacking. And though Depp's character does achieve some level of peace with Mom, the events that follow are shocking in what they represent (though, given Western culture's unhealthy obsessions, hardly surprising).

Mom goes upstairs to bed for the first time in years, and dies. After the authorities inform the family that Mom's corpse will have to be lifted from the house by crane, Depp, terrified of the humiliation this will cause, he says, for her, undertakes with his siblings to burn the house with Mom inside. The end of the film shows Depp and his younger brother (the sisters were dispatched somewhere else) waiting for Lewis to come and take them away in her camper van. What is interesting here is that a male character, Gilbert's brother (played by a very young Leonardo DiCaprio, who was Oscar-nominated for this role), young, impetuous, mentally disabled and often a danger to himself, is allowed to survive and make demands on Depp's character. even while the film-maker kills off the mother.

What does Mom represent? I believe a number of anxieties: various excesses of North American cultures; 'dysfunctional' families and the demands they make on individuals, fear of women, terrifyingly erotic (DiCaprio's character is very attached physically to his mother), but also seen as 'too much'; fear of difference. Her death is highly significant, representing the desire to destroy the sources of such anxieties. The presentation of Mom's predicament as something *she* might have overcome, perhaps by losing some of her weight, or maybe by merely confronting her own traumas and resolving them, just could not have been achieved within this film. Mom was never meant to be a person, a subject: she could only function as a spectacle, an object of our gaze.

Both films raise various questions for me, a fat woman in the audience. How, for example, do other fat women feel about these portrayals of women like us? Is this *really* how others see us, as objects of derision, pity, horror or hatred? Are these the cultural messages written on bodies like mine? I am, I have often been told, a good-looking woman (by Western standards). I am known, apparently, for having a sharp wit, a warm and vivacious personality, an infectious laugh. I know that I am desired sexually. I have also, I believe, made a good many achievements in my life: a number of published works, a Masters degree and other qualifications, two wonderful children (by my standards!). I am artistic, musical, creative and lively, and I love my life. I must promptly reassure the reader that this paragraph is not an attempt to massage my ego. It merely serves, I hope, to give a small indication of the diversity of fat women and to illustrate some of the problems we face as real people, subjects, members of our social communities, in a culture which insists on designating us as objects: a predicament most women find themselves in, but which has particular ramifications for fat women. How am I to live as a fat woman: as a self-directing, active participant in social life, or as a mere object on which others can play out their own fears and fixations? And if my body is used as a repository for other people's anxieties, how does that affect *my* mental health?

Occasionally, Hollywood produces films in which a fat (or at least slightly larger than thin) woman protagonist triumphs over adversity, sometimes finding happiness in romantic love. Sometimes her fat body is an issue within these films, and sometimes not. Examples of such films include *Fried Green Tomatoes at the Whistle-stop Café* and *Dolores Claiborne* (where the lead is taken by actress Kathy Bates), *Hairspray* and *Babycakes* starring Ricki Lake (before she dieted), and *Baghdad Café*. These films show that it is possible for far-sighted film-makers to subvert the unwritten yet dominant codes of Hollywood cinema and reflect real lives a little more. For this to happen more often − and it is significant that I have no examples from the late 1990s − requires enormous determination from such film-makers (and women actors). Perhaps what we really need is more fat women film-makers.

Women are forever conscious of themselves as being watched. Fat women, subjected to unease about their dress sizes as well as the physical signs of their gender, are fully aware that their bodies overflow the boundaries imposed on them by Western cultural and social norms. The ways that fat women perceive themselves will have been shaped by these dominant ideologies. Yet our lived experiences inside our bodies conflict with these cultural demands, and in many ways fat women have the capacity to *resist* such damaging restrictions. Part of my research project will be to find out ways in which we do this. I believe our potential to resist is infinite, especially as we identify the various preoccupations − and their pathological expressions − that pervade Western culture. I think we will find ways, both political and personal, not only of resisting these harmful cultural practices and attitudes, but also of thinking that will allow us to love and care for and respect ourselves as well as others.

As a fat woman watching *Gilbert Grape*, even while feeling

anger at the engineered death of the film's fat character, I found humour in both that plot, and that of the house's foundations being at risk: not because I found Mom's problems amusing in a futile attempt to distance myself from her, but because I recognised that the scenes merely reflected the predictable, transparent and absurd fixations of the film-maker. I was laughing at the *film-maker*, not Mom. It is in such recognitions by women of the foibles of others who, in various positions of power, would author our lives for us, that we can act to transform our world and live our lives as we wish to: nobody's fall-guys.

Walk on the Wide Side

Maxine Molloy

Contrary to popular belief I haven't always been fat. Forty years ago I made my debut weighing a modest 6lb 2oz. Many an oven ready chicken has more meat on it than I did. In fact I suspect I was far less appealing than a freshly plucked chicken. Bald, big nosed even then and with huge, blue veins throbbing visibly beneath papery skin I resembled a baby bird fallen from the nest. And no amount of lovingly knitted matinee jackets and bonnets could disguise my resemblance to a skinned Chihuahua.

The smallest of my mother's five children, I have since more than made up for this insubstantial beginning. Today I tip the scales (on the rare occasions when I can be persuaded to mount them) at about 21 stone. These days the only poultry I bear a resemblance to is a plump, succulent Christmas turkey, mouth-watering and oozing with tasty juices.

For some reason people seem to imagine that I've always been a whopper. Former colleagues found it so difficult to believe that I had ever been slim that I was forced to produce photographic evidence to the contrary. Well I've been fat and I've been thin and let me tell you, fat is better. I've done svelte, I've done slinky, I've done skin and bone. Being thin never made me happy but I will concede that it allowed me to be miserable with a better wardrobe.

I went on my first diet at 11 but I recall being bigger than my contemporaries from about eight onwards. At ten I had size 7 feet and was already able to borrow my older sister's size

10 boutique bargains (this was the swinging 60s). I entered my teens 5′ 9″ tall and two or three stones heavier than my classmates. I felt huge, clumsy and ashamed of my bulk.

What I didn't realise was that I was comparing myself to petite little girls who didn't reach my chest and wouldn't weigh 8 stone fully dressed and carrying bowling balls in their school bags.

Hardly surprising then, that at 17 I flirted with anorexia and managed to get down to nine stone by means of confining my food intake to a meagre slice of bread and one Dairylea cheese triangle per day. About once a week I would allow myself to eat a tin of tomato soup as a special treat. After a couple of years I began to eat a little more but managed to keep my weight constant by swimming five miles a week and walking the three miles home from school every day. It's hard to believe now but so distorted was my body image that I still thought I was a stone overweight.

At university I gained a stone and hovered at around that weight for the next five years, still sporadically dieting and imagining myself to be as swollen and unsightly as a blimp. When I married at 26 my weight gradually crept up to 14½ stone. I spent the next few years alternately losing and gaining weight, all the time hating myself and my body. It was the most miserable period of my life.

I dieted constantly, deluding myself that if I were slimmer everything would be different. I lost weight, I gained it again. If I'd managed to keep off all the weight I ever lost, I'd fit on a key-ring. I tried every crank diet known to humanity and hungrily devoured slimming magazines. I tried the F Plan diet; it gave me wind. The high protein diet gave me bad breath. The Scarsdale gave me the shakes, the cheese diet gave me nightmares. I tried slimming pills which made me hyperactive and paranoid; but on the bright side at least I got the housework done. The low carbohydrate diet gave me constipation and the Cambridge diet gave me an overdraft.

I went to the local Slimming World club, Weight Watchers,

Slimming Magazine club, and Overeaters Anonymous. I've stopped those people who wear badges saying 'Lose weight now, ask me how'.

Gradually, I realised that this cycle of dieting and bingeing was dominating my life. Worse, it was ruining my health and my self-esteem. My diets always failed and I regularly indulged in wild eating binges. I felt a failure and I felt out of control. Food was controlling me. I had finally made the crucial realisation that my problem was not that I was fat, but that I was addicted to food. I had an eating disorder and I would never be happy unless I dealt with it. I began haunting the local library ordering any book I could find that dealt with compulsive eating. In those days there weren't very many but gradually I began to realise that the root of my problem was a lack of self-esteem. This piece of knowledge hit me like a bombshell. How could I love myself if I hated the way I looked? How could I love myself if I spent every waking moment berating myself for my appearance and lack of willpower? More importantly, how could I change unless I accepted myself as I was?

I had never bought myself new clothes, not feeling that I deserved them and always imagining that my current size was only temporary. I tried to survive, and meet the demands of my professional life as a radio producer, by squeezing myself into uncomfortable, restrictive garments and a few larger, charity shop buys. One day I threw out all the old clothes and replaced them with things in my size, promising myself that if I ever got back to a size 12 I would buy myself new ones. Well I haven't replaced them yet, but I do have a wardrobe full of attractive, wearable, well-fitting clothes.

Gradually, I learned to value myself, to appreciate my positive qualities and accept the areas in which I was less than perfect. I realised that I was filled with repressed anger which I controlled by overeating – in fact I eventually came to realise that I managed all my emotions by eating, stuffing down difficult emotions by stuffing down food. I learned how to give those repressed emotions expression and was surprised to discover how much better I felt as a result. One day I realised that I was no longer obsessed with food – with eating it, or not eating it, or dreaming about eating it. About the same time I also discovered that I liked myself exactly as I was.

The process I have summarised in a mere paragraph actually took ten years. Ten long years of soul-searching, extensive reading, sporadic therapy and sheer hard work. Today when I look in the mirror I see a woman with great hair, good skin and a warm smile. An attractive woman whom I like, respect and admire. And if she can't squeeze her arse into a size 12 bikini, or even into a seat on the train, it doesn't detract one iota from any of those qualities.

Where once I hovered in the shadows I now relish the limelight. These days I am happy to wave the banner for us bountiful belles. I've made something of a career defending the rights of the generously proportioned. I've even appeared on TV from time to time when they want the services of an articulate large lady to talk about size issues. Well I'm definitely a large lass and if articulate means 'never shuts up' I am guilty as charged.

One of the most pleasant discoveries I have made since accepting my size is that men crave curves. Far from fancying Kate Moss and her skinny sisters, your average guy likes his girl to have a bit of padding.

However, a bountiful babe does need to be wary of the chubby chaser. Mr CC is a man who's never got over being weaned. He doesn't want an equal partner or a relationship of mutual respect. He wants his mummy. He wants you to bounce him on your knee and burp him.

Such men are easily spotted. It's not just the thumb-sucking that gives it away, or their obsessive fascination with breasts. It's their reverent worship of female flesh in large quantities. You wouldn't believe the number of men who, when I enquired why they prefer larger ladies, have told me that they fantasise about 'getting lost in the folds'. While I love to be appreciated this hardly seems healthy. What's more they don't appear to realise that I might find such an image less than appealing. I always think it makes me sound like Jabba the Hut and the hopeful suitor sound as insignificant and irritating as a mosquito.

Fortunately there are a refreshingly large proportion of men who just want to worship at the altar of womanhood. And I've always been a great believer in religious freedom.

Personally I tend to prefer my men on the bountiful side. I want to let rip in bed without worrying about injuries. I want someone whose knee I can sit on occasionally and clothes I can borrow. Or vice versa if we're feeling adventurous. I want someone who doesn't make us look like refugees from a McGill postcard when we go to the beach. Someone with whom I can share a seesaw, without running the risk of launching him into orbit like a human catapult.

My current partner is 6′ 7″ and built like a whole row of brick outhouses. If we go for a swim at the beach, concerned onlookers telephone Greenpeace. If we take a walk in the park children flock round, mistaking us for a couple of recently landed hot air balloons. Unless we're careful we can block out the sun. If ever a match was made in heaven, it's ours.

Being larger than average is always good for a laugh. Several years ago I went to Paris in the springtime with the man of my dreams, as he called himself. When we arrived in the city of lurve I had an unforgettable experience which sent my heart pounding, my temperature soaring and left me thoroughly breathless and damp with sweat. Unfortunately, the cause of this little death was not a romantic indoor interlude with my beloved but a bout of exercise of an entirely different kind. Although it did involve the earth moving. No doubt everyone finds climbing the steps up to Sacré Coeur in Montmartre a bit of a trek, but when we leaned on the ancient marble parapet for support, we both felt it shift dramatically under our weight. We leapt back in horrified disbelief, but it had definitely moved. It might have stood for over a century and withstood the pounding feet of millions of visitors but two overfed Brits had nearly ended all that. We could picture the headlines: 'Sacré Bleu! Ten ton tourists topple Sacré Coeur'. So we hot-footed it sharpish. As sharpish as two out of breath couch-potatoes who felt as though they had just walked up Everest were capable of. And although we expected to be pursued round every corner by irate gendarmes muttering Gallic oaths and brandishing their pistols, we managed to make a clean getaway.

But unfortunately, being a big girl isn't always a barrel of laughs. When I was asked to write this essay I was due to be admitted to hospital for what plastic surgeons call a rhinoplasty and what the rest of us call a nose job. If you find it ironic that I have achieved size acceptance but cannot extend this process to include loving my nose, let me emphasise that my reasons for seeking surgery were not purely cosmetic. Eight years ago I was hurrying to work along a Cardiff street on a chilly, winter morning when I tripped on a broken paving stone. Unable to get my hands out of my coat pockets in time, I went down like a felled tree. I hit the pavement face first and my nose snapped like a twig. When it finally healed I was left with a bump which would make Barry McGuigan envious, a crushed nostril and permanent breathing problems. I first enquired about the possibility of having it corrected more than two years ago and was put on the waiting list of a London hospital one year later.

Now let me remind you that I weigh 21 stone. A fairly substantial weight and not one that is easily overlooked. Naturally I had read articles in the press about larger people being refused operations or asked to lose weight. And since my size is self evident to even the most casual observer I naively assumed that it was not a factor in my case. But not so.

The day of my scheduled operation I was admitted and processed and only then was it mentioned to me that the anaesthetist *might* be concerned about my size. There then followed a three-hour wait during which I was quizzed and consulted by various medical personnel about my general health, my previous operations and, of course, my weight. I was beginning to get a very bad feeling about it all.

Eventually I was informed that the anaesthetist had refused to do my operation. Apparently the type of anaesthetic used in nose operations is different from the usual sort and involves more risk. I was informed that my Body Mass Index was 44 and that 'normal people' are 25. I was described as 'morbidly obese', a term which, as a comedy writer, I found both insulting and ironic. I was told that when a fat person lies down the bottom third of the lungs collapse, making ventilation during an operation more difficult. I was assured that we are more difficult to intubate because of fat in the throat. The picture of me which was being painted did not relate *at all* to the happy, healthy and active woman I know I am. And although they didn't tell me in words of one syllable that I was a freak who ought to be ashamed of herself, that was the message I got.

Finally, the consultant said 'I suppose you're feeling rather depressed about all this.' Images of bulls being taunted with red rags and camels' spines snapping under the weight of final straws filled my imagination. I summoned up all my dignity, composure and eloquence and explained to her that rather than depression I felt the fiery lava of righteous anger coursing through my veins. She visibly whitened as I reminded her that it is not possible to weigh 21 stone secretly. That even the most well-fitting clothes cannot disguise or conceal such a size. She seemed to shrink and wither as I reminded her that I had been this size for the past ten years, and certainly weighed the same at my outpatient's appointment 13 months previously. She could only nod her head in mute agreement when I pointed out that if my size was an issue now it must certainly have been 13 months ago. And she could offer no explanation as to why such a significant and obvious factor was not brought to my attention at that time so I could have taken some action prior to the proposed operating date. Finally, after I had waited for her answer for what seemed like aeons, she managed to mumble 'That's a fair point.'

Eventually we agreed that I would lose some weight in order to have the operation. At first they wanted me to lose 10 stone, but I argued that they must perform operations all the time on people who are not their ideal weight. We agreed that I would lose five or six stone and then be reassessed. This probably means that I will have to wait another year for the procedure. So here I am, perfectly happy with my size, but dieting so I can have an operation. Fortunately, I am highly motivated so I'm not finding it too difficult. I am also finding it a useful way of channelling my, as yet undiminished, anger. Still, looking on the bright side, I can always put it back on again afterwards.

If nothing else, life as a large lass is character building. It has sharpened my sense of humour and honed my assertiveness skills. I've also learned that beauty, or its opposite, is very much in the eye of the beholder. One person's morbidly obese is another's pleasantly plump. And over the years I've come to realise that there is one section of the population who can be totally non-judgemental about those of us who are broader in the beam. It's true what they say about babes and sucklings: many a pearl of wisdom has fallen from their chubby lips – and you can always count on a child to tell you the truth. My seven-year-old niece, Eve, dispenses gems of wisdom and insight so regularly that she could take up a career as an agony aunt. Comforting euphemisms and empty platitudes are not part of her vocabulary; she is direct, straightforward and matter of fact. When her goldfish died she responded to my sister's attempts to assure her that they had 'gone to a lovely place' by announcing 'I'm sorry to tell you this, but they didn't go to a lovely place, they went in the bin.' Thus giving my sister a lesson on overcoming denial and facing bereavement that Oprah would have been proud of.

Perhaps my brother and his wife knew a thing or two when they named her after the first woman. In her innocence Eve sees things as they really are, unclouded by prejudice, preconception or peer pressure. Although I might be outsize, obese, buxom or gross to the world at large, in Eve's eyes I am 'lovely and cuddly'. When she climbs onto my knee for a story there's also room to accommodate Postman Pat, Thomas the Tank Engine and as many members of her cuddly toy collection as she cares to bring. She regards my lap as a soft and welcoming place of refuge and my bountiful bosom as a well-upholstered cushion. If she's feeling sleepy she can stretch out for a cuddle and when she's in a livelier mood I am her personal bouncy castle.

Although it may have taken me half a lifetime of dieting and self-loathing to realise that there is life after size 18, my niece seems to have learned this lesson at a remarkably early age. Her wholehearted appreciation of my proportions has helped me to be proud of my size and made me realise how powerful and destructive stereotypes can be. With Eve's help I have learned to appreciate my curves. Society may urge me to conform, disregard my femininity and try to ignore me, but Eve simply believes there is more of me to love. And I have no intention of disagreeing with her. In fact, she has got me thinking about the advantages of being ample.

Although it's all too easy to accept the daily brainwashing that tries to convince us to conform, a resourceful woman can easily discover ways in which her size can work for her. I always get a seat to myself on public transport, for instance, and so get to pass my journey in relative luxury.

Restaurant managers extend a warm welcome when I book a table and I receive the most attentive and sycophantic service. The only exceptions being those establishments that offer 'all you can eat' buffets to whom the arrival of a couple of hungry heavyweights can threaten bankruptcy.

Nobody ever tries to queue-jump in my presence and bar staff can't pretend they haven't noticed me. Hard theatre and cinema seats aren't quite so uncomfortable when you bring your own padding. I'm well insulated in the winter and become very popular when there's a draught in the room because skinny people can keep warm by snuggling up to me.

In the summer when I cool off in the pool I am extra buoyant and have natural water wings. And nobody ever, ever bothers to ask me 'Does my bum look big in this?'

Although I might have written the above list with my tongue firmly in my cheek, it does demonstrate the fact that to appreciate the benefits of being bulky you just have to exercise your lateral thinking skills. More important, I have found that if you want to be taken seriously in a masculine dominated environment, size is a definite advantage. In the boardroom qualities like power, bulk and the ability to dominate space are essential qualities. Although a slim woman can develop these attributes a big one has a huge head start.

If your size makes you self-conscious, developing a more positive attitude can transform an anxiety into an asset. Being highly visible means that you can't be ignored. A bountiful babe can hold the floor at business meetings, command the attention of shop assistants and be the belle of the ball. Most of us crave attention, being bigger than average ensures we get it. And once you've got it, flaunt it. Don't ever let anyone tell you less is more. Nothing exceeds like excess and you can't have too much of a good thing. It can be fun, it can be funny, it can be frustrating, but life in the fat lane is never boring. Down these lean streets a woman must walk who is not herself lean. Why not join me for a walk on the wide side?

The Other 'F' Word
Fat, Physical Correctness and the Body Police

Maggie Millar

In the early sixties when I was aboard an Italian ship sailing for England I looked a little like one of the most popular movie stars of the day, Sophia Loren – she of the voluptuous body, bold eyes and full lips – the epitome of eternal Woman. It was a look I cultivated and the stewards on the ship used to call out 'Ciao, Sophia!' as I passed by.

There was a wonderful programme about Loren on television not long ago. Looking at her I realised that if she were to arrive in Hollywood looking for work today, she would be told to go away, have a nose job, and lose fifteen kilos; that magnificent womanly body would actually prevent her from working. and the world would be denied her considerable talent. The same would apply to Marilyn Monroe who wore a size 16 dress in *Some Like it Hot*.

When I was breaking hearts on the *Fairsky* back then, I used to be a size 12–14; I'm now a size 18–20. This is as a result of a number of factors, not the least of which is having been a 'career dieter' for some thirty years. (Other factors include my gender, age, metabolism, and, most importantly, inherited body shape and size.)

I have been thinking recently, as preparation for writing this piece, of all the diets I have been on in my life. One of the first that I remember was when I was at RADA during one of the worst English winters on record (not an easy thing for an Australian to come to terms with!). I was living on a scholarship and the rather stodgy canteen food was very cheap and very comforting – lots of steak and kidney pudding, chips, roasts with three veg and gravy, steamed puds, etc. The teaching staff had seen my girth expand a little – not a huge amount, but enough to prevent me from filling the physically correct requirements of the current ideal. (Twiggy had arrived by then, so I was in big trouble!) I was sent to a Harley Street doctor who specialised in rapid weight loss for his many clients.

There was a constant stream of women from all over London beating a track to his elegant suite of rooms; he was obviously doing very nicely thank you. We were put on an 800 calorie a day diet, and on our daily visits to the clinic were injected in the buttocks (right cheek one day, left the next) with a serum which was purported to contain the urine of pregnant women. I don't know how true this was, but apparently something in this substance was supposed to cause the metabolism to speed up. I suppose when you're desperate you'll believe anything. I certainly did lose weight rapidly (and got a very sore bum), but of course the weight went back on in no time at all once I started feeding myself adequately.

Since that time, I have 'done' just about every diet that's ever been invented, from the Israeli Army diet (did the Israeli Army *really* exist on two days of cheese?) to the egg and grapefruit diet (nine hard-boiled eggs a day can have a disastrous effect on one's social life).

I have spent countless dollars on exercise equipment, *hours* exercising at gyms, lifting weights, running on treadmills (getting nowhere!) and doing boring aerobics with less and less effect as I have got older. I have fasted, lived on fruit juice, eaten weird diet 'biscuits', taken amphetamines and ghastly powdered diet supplements, even sucked on cough lollies as an appetite suppressant. Thankfully, I have never taken laxatives, or induced vomiting in order to lose weight.

For virtually all of my career, I have been at war with my body; on the yo-yo diet treadmill in order to gain a certain role, to earn enough money, to have my abilities recognised. (While I do not believe, nor ever have, that I was 'owed' a living – especially in a profession with such a high unemployment rate – nevertheless I was one of the minority who worked more often than not.) On more than one occasion I have been told, 'Lose a bit of weight, and you're a serious contender for this role.' And then I'd try another diet.

The effects of this long-term abuse of my digestive system – not to mention my sense of self-worth – are numerous as I've said: three or five sizes larger than when I started out, a very intolerant digestive system, depression, and for the last couple of years, since I have overcome my clinical depression, what I suspect is Chronic Fatigue Syndrome. Hardly surprising really!

I have, however, finally learned from these experiences. I no longer berate myself for not sticking to a diet; I haven't dieted for some eight years now, and my weight has stayed pretty much the same. I can't begin to tell you how truly liberating it has been to get off that treadmill. I can now enjoy my husband's bacon and eggs every Sunday without feeling guilty. (I don't mean I eat his as well as mine; he cooks!) I have learned to accept the natural changes in my body as I grow older. And I have had to confront the deeper implications of the current societal expectations upon women to be thin in order to be successful, sexy or simply okay.

When I worked in *Prisoner: Cell Block H*, playing 'top dog' Marie Winter, I was surrounded by a cast of talented women who were all shapes, sizes and ages. Because the show was set in a prison, and therefore beyond the pale of 'normal' society, we were permitted to appear without the usual distortions of the feminine typically seen on commercial television, films and in magazines. Another TV series which was set behind high walls – *Brides of Christ* – also featured a cast of non-stereotypical women, apart from the two leads. Nuns don't live in 'normal' society either, so they too can forgo what I call the Physically Correct Imperative (PCI). Despite their great talent, very few of these women have been seen on our screens in other productions; the PCI still reigns supreme.

For over thirty years I worked in an industry in which as a

general rule, and with very few notable exceptions, a woman is only considered worth employing if her boobs are forever perky, her face forever young, and she has 'buns of steel'! In the entertainment industry – in Australia at any rate – the size of one's waistline is more important than the size of one's talent (except for comedians – but then fat women are not to be taken seriously).

During the course of my work, I have both studied and portrayed a wide variety of people. It has therefore been necessary to understand why people behave the way they do and, most importantly, not to judge them in any way whatsoever. This was particularly true of the character I played in *Prisoner: Cell Block H* – a woman seemingly without any redeeming characteristics at all!

That necessity to suspend moral judgement has enabled me to empathise with people who are often the targets of moral outrage and reprobation from those among us who fit certain current ideals – none more so than those who are not considered physically correct. (And if you think the Thought Police have had an impact, I can assure you that the Body Police leave them for dead.)

For some years now – in fact virtually since leaving the acting profession – my curiosity has been engaged by the phenomenon of fat phobia and related issues: dieting, body dissatisfaction, eating disorders, etc, all of which are obviously connected.

My involvement with these issues came about as a direct result of their impact in my own life: ie my capacity to earn a living. When I could no longer stave off the effects of being a career dieter and a 'certain age' – and of course, like millions of other women, I blamed my lack of 'willpower' for losing the battle – my livelihood, which up till then had been reasonably adequate, became highly problematic. It therefore became necessary for my own psychic survival to come to terms with the current obsession with physical correctness which has impacted so directly on my life. As a result, the personal for me has become hugely political.

As Carl Jung said: '...if the connection between the personal problem and the larger contemporary event is discerned and understood, it brings release from the loneliness of the purely personal, and the subjective problem is magnified into a general question of our society. In this way, the personal problem acquires a dignity it lacked hitherto.'[1]

And I can absolutely vouch for that. In fact I remember vividly the tears I shed when I discerned in the very depths of my being the connection between my own dilemma (rapidly diminishing offers of work), the current obsession with the 'perfect' – read 'distorted' – female body and the profound denial of the feminine principle in our society. Because that, I believe, is the *real* issue here: the negation of the power and importance of this principle in Western society; and that is why 'big' women cannot be acknowledged or celebrated. They epitomise that power; they are the physical manifestation of the female. 'Notice me, I'm a *woman*!' they say. (Not a pouting androgynous adolescent stick-insect!)

When I no longer fitted the PCI, I was faced with a serious dilemma. What do I do now? The following years were deeply painful for me. I suffered from clinical depression and I realised after much soul-searching (literally – I was seeing a Jungian therapist) that the industry in which I had worked for so long was in fact not good for *my* soul: that innate feminine self which I was only just beginning to understand.

I had been asked to talk to 900 girls at a large private girls' school in Melbourne about body image, popular culture and dieting. The teachers were concerned about the growing incidence of problematic eating patterns and eating disorders in the school.

I began to do some research. I read all I could. I talked to various professionals. I ran a couple of focus groups with women friends of all ages and I talked with women in the entertainment industry. It became abundantly clear that this issue impacts on the lives of women of all ages, shapes and backgrounds. And it's no different eight years later. In fact it's a whole lot worse.

I did my presentation at the girls' school, and much to my surprise, received a standing ovation. The teacher who initially asked me to speak told a colleague, word spread, and I have continued to talk to school students ever since.

I believe that if the whole person is not considered when we address this issue, we might as well not bother. It's about so much more than counting calories and the 'right' amount of exercise, about 'good' and 'bad' foods, or the latest scientific study into why some people are fatter than others. I have therefore devised a series of workshops and seminars which enable women to untangle some of the threads which contribute to poor body/self-image, and have some fun at the same time! These include:

i) distinguishing between internal and external attitudes,
ii) looking critically at media images,
iii) investigating statements concerning health, size, weight, etc,
iv) modifying self-talk and developing a more balanced perspective,
v) making time for inner needs, and
vi) most importantly, laughing, moving and enjoying the body, whatever size, age or shape: feeling the power *in* the body, as opposed to the power *of* the body.

I use videos, images on overheads, discussion, information sheets (or 'takeaways'). I point out the misinformation related to fat, weight, women and health which is part of the received wisdom of our society. For example, contrary to popular belief:

* A certain amount of fat – at *least* 18–20% – is absolutely necessary for health in women.
* Being fat can have health benefits.[2]
* There is no universally accepted, scientifically validated definition of 'overweight' or 'obesity'.[3]
* Some studies show that fat women – even at the upper

end of the scale – live longer and have fewer health problems than thin women.[4]

* Hypertension in fat people is often caused by the attitudes of society, especially the health and medical professions.[5]

* Fat people have the same health rights as thin people.

* Height/weight charts, which some professionals still use, are based on an unrepresentative sample and were in fact originated by an insurance company in the USA.[6]

* On its own a sedentary lifestyle will not lead to 'obesity' unless the individual is genetically predisposed.[7]

* The Body Mass Index (BMI) is a totally ineffective device for measuring health (it showed that a group of physically tuned American gridiron players were unhealthily overweight!).[8]

* In the words of psychotherapist Dr Margaret Sheridan: '... a message that was designed for middle-aged, overweight, smoking, boozing men has been taken up with a vengeance by young women.'[9]

In my workshops I use drama exercises, stories, drawing, music, meditation, movement and laughter. I always have a candle burning, and some fragrant oils. I have a mascot: Beryl the Ballerina, a statue of a very large woman in a white tutu *en pointe*! I find that a multi-faceted approach is most effective – food for the body, mind, heart and soul.

It always helps to have a good laugh, and any of the French and Saunders videos fill that bill superbly, as does the work of the wonderful Australian comedian Magda Szubanski (Magda played the appalling farmer's wife in the *Babe* movies).

The push for physical correctness is also largely driven by money: market forces determine to some extent the prevailing social attitudes towards large people – especially women – despite the loud protestations from advertisers that they are 'only reflecting public opinion'. Imagine the effect on the 'market' if every woman in the Western world woke up tomorrow feeling perfectly okay about her appearance. The diet, cosmetic, fitness, health and beauty industries would cease to exist, and plastic surgeons would no longer be able to afford their Mercs and Beamers.

Jungian therapist and writer Marion Woodman, in her book *The Owl was a Baker's Daughter*, writes of the devaluation and distortion of the feminine as now being manifested in the fat woman and her exact opposite: the woman suffering from anorexia nervosa: '...in the Western countries...the feminine has been devalued for centuries and is now profoundly distorted. In our culture where the feminine is denigrated...fatness, not sex, is a taboo...and [fatness] has taken on evil and immoral overtones.'

The ridicule, hostility, and moral superiority usually manifested towards fat women bears witness in a very concrete way to Western society's rejection of the feminine. The fat woman receives no sympathy or understanding whatsoever, and is often judged as lazy, out of control, greedy – morally defective, in other words, whereas her size is more often a combination of many factors, not the least of which is constant dieting. And even if she uses food as a substitute for other hungers in her life, what right does anyone have to judge her? Let alone refuse her medical treatment, as has happened on some occasions.

We still believe that if a woman is fat, and therefore, apparently, open to such vilification, it is *entirely* her own fault. Otherwise she would have tried harder, she would have lost 'the weight', she would have discarded her excess flesh, no matter what it cost her. She would have more control over her 'appetites'. In the words of 'obesity' specialist Dr David Schlund, 'fat loathing' has become 'the last permissible social prejudice. Most people would never use a racial or ethnic slur in public, but clients tell me that people come up to them all the time and call them fat slobs.'[10]

On the other hand the woman (or often young girl) who suffers from anorexia nervosa receives much sympathy – as indeed she should – and many women grudgingly admire the frightening control shown by the anorectic, whose refusal to nourish herself, in many cases to the point of death, causes such devastation to herself, her family and friends.

Fear of fat is endemic in this society. Despite the ever-increasing volume of evidence that diets don't work and cause many more problems than they purport to solve, despite the biological necessity for fat on the female body (oestrogen is stored in fatty tissue, something which many women forget), despite even '... the evidence irrefutably accumulated in repeated studies that fat people are sexier, and want more sex more often than thin people'[11] we still refuse to let go of the lie and believe we should hate and reject the very thing that makes us female.

Why? Why do we hang on to this fear of fat with such tenacity? Is it merely because we are bombarded daily with anti-fat messages from so many different places. or is it something more profound? Is it because we still believe that lack of control in the female, be it the body, the psyche or the emotions, is greatly to be feared?

Control and repression of the feminine – is that what this is really about? Why else, in order to be valued and rewarded, must women exercise the most rigid control of the personal feminine, their own bodies? (And those women who are seen as not controlling their errant female flesh – fat women – become our society's pariahs.)

What does this deep-seated fear of fat say about the un-willingness of so many women to rebel against these debilitating strictures? What are we so afraid of?

It is rejection. Rejection by 'society', by employers, our peers, our children, by men. Yet in order to be 'acceptable', we ourselves must collude in the rejection of our own diverse female realities. It's no wonder, in the face of such a cruel double-bind, that so many women and ever younger girls are manifesting eating 'disorders'. (And what a neat little euphemism that is.)

'But fat is unhealthy!' the Body Police cry, and of course too much of it *can* be; we all know that. I would ask, however, how much is too much for whom (most studies on 'obesity' and health have been carried out on men), and what other issues are involved? Let's face it, too much of anything is bad for your health: stress, thinness, exercise, alcohol, anger, testosterone, libido, coffee, smoking, leisure, work, control... I could go on and on. Health is an enormously complex matter comprising emotional, mental and spiritual – as well as physical – well-being, a fact that seems to elude the Body Police, who seem intent on making life a misery for anyone who does not fit the PCI.

Marion Woodman has asserted that: 'Twentieth-century women have been living for centuries in a male oriented culture which has kept them unconscious of their own feminine principle... they have unknowingly accepted male values – goal oriented lives, compulsive drivenness and concrete bread which fails to nourish their feminine mystery. Their unconscious femininity rebels and manifests in some somatic form.'[12]

Another Jungian therapist, storyteller and best-selling author Clarissa Pinkola Estés, writes: 'A woman's issues of soul cannot be treated by carving her into a more acceptable form as defined by an unconscious culture... When we lose touch with the instinctive psyche, we live in a semi-destroyed state and images and powers that are natural to the feminine are not allowed full development.'[13]

Can we even imagine a society in which the feminine in *all* its aspects is celebrated; where a diversity of female shapes, sizes and ages appear in films, TV shows and magazines; where women are affirmed and given kudos just as they are; where the female body does not have to be constantly fought and tamed (ie starved, cut, stitched, tightened, enhanced, smoothed, plasticised, etc) but is free to wobble and flop and droop, manifesting its natural progressions and changes; where women dance and swim and move and are fully sensual and exultantly sexual, whatever their size or shape or age; where each mother instils in her daughter a fierce pride and joy in her own natural inherited female shape and sex?

One woman alone cannot change the current dis-empowering culture; but she can change her own attitude towards herself, thereby minimising the effect of harmful projections. 'She can do this by reclaiming her own unique physicality, and . . . by not forsaking the joy of her natural body, by not purchasing the popular illusion that happiness is only bestowed on those of a certain configuration or age, by not waiting or holding back to do anything, and by taking back her real life, and living at full bore, all stops out. This dynamic self-acceptance and self-esteem are what begins to change attitude in the culture.'[14]

Ladies, it's *time*. Time to say *no* to commandments which tell us: Thou shalt not be large, unruly, loud, loose, floppy or old! Thou shalt not be thyself. Thou shalt not let thyself go! (And we all know that if you can't let yourself go, you can't let yourself . . . do the opposite. Hardly a recipe for a sensational sex life!)

Let us turn off the television sets, boycott the magazines, refuse to buy the products, and stop going to the films until they show us in all our wonderful diversity.

Let us stop the diets, give up plastic surgery, swim and dance in public places – even if we're large, or old (or both!), demand gorgeous clothes for all ages, shapes and sizes, and generally put ourselves about.

Let us ignore the cultural imperative that tells us to reject our own deepest soul, and our own myriad physical realities. Let us give permission for girl children to be *children*, for middle-aged women to expand, and for old women to show by their lines and wrinkles, that they have actually lived full, productive and interesting lives.

Personally, I look forward to becoming the large, unruly, colourful old woman I suspect is waiting at the end of the hall. And if others don't like her, well frankly my dears, I don't give a damn! I'll be too busy enjoying myself.

NOTES

1. Jung, Carl Gustav, *The Essential Jung,* ed. Anthony Storr (Princeton University Press, Princeton, 1983)
2. Martin, Alison & Hood, Cassandra: Introduction to *The Healthy Mind & Body Chart* (Adelaide Nutrition Care, Adelaide, 1996)
3. *Ibid*
4. Ernsberger & Haskew, 'Rethinking Obesity' (*Journal of Obesity & Weight Reduction,*Vol. 6, No. 2, 1987)
5. Bovey, Shelley, *The Forbidden Body:Why Being Fat Is Not a Sin* (Pandora/HarperCollins, London, 1994)
6. Martin & Hood, Introduction to *The Healthy Mind & Body Chart*
7. Dr Joe Prioetto, Director, Centre for the Study of Obesity, *The Australian* Weekend Magazine, 1996
8. Martin & Hood, Introduction to *The Healthy Mind & Body Chart* (Adelaide Nutrition Care, Adelaide, 1996)
9 Millar, M, *Caring for Health* (Report on NSW Ministerial Summit on Eating Disorders, 1996)
10. Schlund, Dr David, *Cleo* Magazine, May 1998
11. Klein, Professor Richard, *Eat Fat* (Pantheon Books, New York, 1996)
12. Woodman, Marion, *The Owl Was A Baker's Daughter* (Inner City Books, Canada, 1980)
13. Estés, Clarissa Pinkola, *Women Who Run with the Wolves* (Ballantine Books, NY, 1995)
14. *Ibid*

Style is an Attitude – Not a Size

Janice Bhend

I still do not quite understand why I felt the need to try and change society's attitude to size, but it seems as if, all my life, I have been on some kind of mission, a search for the truth behind a big, fat lie that larger people are worthless, unhealthy, lazy, stupid and greedy. I knew I wasn't any of those things and I was certainly born for the part. I've been large all my life, a bouncing 9lb 10oz baby, a chubby child, a tubby teenager when, in the swinging sixties, it was only acceptable to be Twiggy shaped. I do not remember suffering victimisation at school, though perhaps time has drawn a discreet veil over any unpleasantness. I do remember the ignominy of the school medical, when in our navy knickers we lined up to be weighed. That agony only served to ensure that in adult life I never even considered joining a slimming club, I was not prepared to accept any further humiliation through public weighing. I do recall making a conscious decision quite early on, that I did not want to commit myself to a lifetime of censored eating and deprivation in order to become and maintain a fashionable size. I concluded that I was one of nature's more generously built specimens, and tried to conduct myself accordingly, without apology.

From the perspective of more than 35 years, I understand now that my career in journalism, and particularly the almost five years with *YES!*, has been for me a kind of exorcism. In the words of a popular old song, I tried to 'accentuate the positive and eliminate the negative' and prove that I could succeed and be happy not despite my size but because of it. Like the curate's egg 'it was good, in parts'.

My first step along the path to further enlightenment came in the early sixties when I went for an interview for a job as junior in the fashion department of *Woman's Own*, then THE women's weekly magazine. The Fashion Editor, a scary person in sunglasses, a navy coat-dress and matching hat, who I later realised hid her insecurities beneath this uncompromising uniform, offered me the job. I had come home.

Magazines seemed to fulfil for me every single part of my creative soul. Always a people-person, I loved the excitement of never knowing what was going to happen next, or who would arrive through the office door. Joanna Lumley was a regular visitor, a much sought-after young model. I was enthralled by the clothes and used to make sketches of them as a record for features before delivering them back to manufacturers in a suitcase by bus. I got to know the rag trade inside out and loved the razzmatazz of it all in London's fashion centre behind Oxford Street. I was asked to call some clothes in for a *Woman's Own* party which was to form the basis of a feature. Personalities of the day came in for fittings – heady stuff – but there was a snag. The only thing I could find to wear myself was a rather sedate black dress, all that was on offer in size 16 that was halfway acceptable, among the Crimplene numbers deemed suitable for larger women.

I progressed in five years, through all areas of the fashion department, answering readers' letters, booking the well-known photographers of the day, David Bailey and Terence Donovan, and models like Jean Shrimpton, Tanya Mallet and Celia Hammond. During my very first shoot as an assistant I burnt the dress with a too-hot iron, a lesson learned and remembered – always iron the back of the garment first, just in case!

Eventually, with the arrival of and encouragement from a new fashion editor, Jane Read, a big girl herself and an inspiration to me, I became a fashion writer. Combining my love of photography and clothes with my joy in the English language created what seemed to me then the perfect job, except for one thing – I still couldn't find the clothes I wanted, to fit. I longed to be able to wear Courrèges boots and a white mini dress, but always had to make do with a compromise. A Vidal Sassoon style bob and pale pink lipstick, along with some snappy shoes, helped to give me an approximation of the look of the moment.

I was offered a job on *Woman & Home*, and joined the magazine just before I got married, in 1966. Shortly after, when *Woman & Home* was merged with *Everywoman*, I became Assistant Fashion Editor on *Woman's Weekly*. Part of the remit was to be responsible for writing and photographing the Over 40 Club column. It wasn't an age, but a size thing, aimed at women whose hips measured 40 inches or over! It was a partnership made in heaven. I tracked down all the information there was to be had about plus size clothes, my enthusiasm showed through and the column became a highly popular part of the magazine. When Britain went over to metric measurements I pointed out that the column would now need to be called the 'Over 101.6 Club' and invented a new name, Sizewise. My pen name, Caroline Hunt, was inherited from a long-dead journalist, and had been kept for the sake of continuity. Caroline and I wrote the column for 26 years, organising Large is Lovely model competitions for readers, and from time to time, Sizewise Specials – eight-page pull-outs incorporating all aspects of difficult-to-find clothes, with items for extra-tall and shorter women, older and less able bodied ones too. I was especially proud of the photo-shoot I did with a woman in a wheelchair. I felt very strongly that fashion should not be reserved for the young, fit and slim, but was something that ought to be enjoyed by everyone.

In my capacity as a size 'expert' I was asked to appear on many TV and radio programmes, and did several for Thames TV's *Afternoon Plus* with Mary Parkinson and Nancy Roberts, a big, bold American woman, way ahead of her time, who wrote the book *Breaking all the Rules*. It dawned on me, when recording these programmes, that many larger women suffered from what I began to think of as the '*Yes-but*' syndrome. The dialogue with the audience would go something like this: Q: 'Why don't "they" make clothes to fit me?' A: 'Well, of course "they" do, I feature them regularly in Sizewise.' Q: '*Yes, but* I want dungarees, where can I find them?' A: 'I know just the company for you!' Q: '*Yes, but* do they do them in yellow?' A: 'I'm sure they do.' Q: '*Yes, but* I expect they are very expensive, I couldn't possibly afford them.' It seemed to me that over and over again, women wanted to blame anyone but themselves for why they couldn't look and feel fashionable. After all, I'd more or less managed it, by using my initiative, and Nancy certainly had, so why couldn't they? Almost without exception, none of those women in day-time TV audiences had made any effort with their hair, make-up or accessories, things that don't depend on size for effect. It was as if they couldn't give themselves 'permission' to look good until they were slim and conforming to society's expectations of them.

After the first of my two sons was born in 1969 I became a freelance, continuing my work for *Woman's Weekly*, but taking on other commissions from specialist magazines like *Choice* and *Saga*, carrying through my theme of fashion for all, whatever age or size. In those days most media folk believed older women, like larger ones, came from a different planet and were amazed, for instance, when we did a fashion show for Central TV and put a 60-year-old in jeans! I did personality interviews too, and met some fascinating people.

While on holiday in the West Country with my family I met someone else who had a profound effect on me. Margaret Peters was almost quadraplegic, yet an athlete who had won medals at the Disabled Olympics for throwing the javelin and who could swim for miles. I persuaded her to give me an interview, subsequently used in *Woman's Weekly*. Margaret said something which I have always remembered, 'It's not what you can't do, but what you can that counts.' I applied that to size. There can be no doubt that being large in our Western world is a social disability. People regard you as 'having let yourself go'. It's the last great permissible prejudice because your size is perceived as being all your own fault – 'You could lose weight after all, if you'd just make the effort.' If only it were really that simple. There are as many reasons for being large as there are large people, but if you simply give up and act like a victim, I reasoned, society treats you as just that. Margaret's totally positive attitude towards her limitations really made me think.

During my career I have been involved with several magazines aimed at the plus size market. The first never happened – a change at board level killed the project before it had begun. I was involved briefly with a very glossy magazine, *Cachet*, which had a short and troubled life, closing down after producing just two issues, then I met Eleanor Graham. She was acting as PR to Carole Shaw, Editor and founder of *BBW* (Big Beautiful Woman) magazine in America. She was in the UK trying to find a British publisher to bring out *BBW* here. Carole's mission was not a success with the sceptical British publishing industry, but after she had returned to the States, Eleanor decided she'd try to do it herself. As Assistant Editor I helped her launch the bi-monthly *Extra Special* in 1986 – the same year that the German magazine *Prima* launched here and changed the British magazine industry for ever. Unlike *Prima*, however, *Extra Special* was run on a shoestring, but was relatively successful with one third of its print run being sold through Evans stores. After two and a half years, Eleanor sold the title, it was relaunched as a monthly, then closed down two issues later. We never knew why, although I suspect it was due to lack of advertising.

After *Extra Special* came *Pretty Big*, a subscription only magazine which I was asked to contribute to, but by then I was planning my own project. I wanted to produce a directory of plus size fashion shops. Ask any large woman why she wants to lose weight and she'll tell you it's because she can't find any clothes to fit. I also knew that many small businesses had begun with high hopes that they could provide the kind of clothes larger women said they wanted, only to close down again rather smartly, due to lack of custom. So I began, with the help of my elder son, a computer wizard, to compile a database, which I intended to launch as a directory and sell by mail order. I sent out a questionnaire, via friendly shops and mail order companies, and had a good response: this was something that was definitely needed. During this time too, I joined forces with a plus size model agency and we ran two workshops in London. Big Day Out proved to be very successful. We had discussion groups, talks from experts and a professional fashion show. The large women who came loved meeting others like themselves and discovering how many of us have the same problems and different ways of solving them.

Meanwhile, back in magazine land, a photographer with whom I had worked many times over the years, wanted to start our own magazine. I was less than enthusiastic; I already knew the pitfalls. He talked me and a designer friend of his into producing a 'dummy', a prototype of how the magazine would look. We took it to a distributor, who showed it to W.H. Smith. They liked it and agreed to take it, so suddenly it became a real possibility. I thought up the title as a reference to *Extra Special* to remind readers of the magazine they had loved and lost – *YES!* stands for You're Extra Special, and is also the most positive word in the English language. As this was to be a totally positive magazine about size, it seemed appropriate. My SpecialSize directory became an integral and eventually much loved part of the product. We found ourselves mustering our own small resources, having once again failed to find a publishing company to back us, and hosting a launch party in September 1993.

Sales and response were initially good. *This Morning* did a short film about us; we appeared on *Jim'll Fix It*, arranging for a young, big girl to be a model for the day; I gave interviews to most of the daily and weekend press and many more radio and TV programmes. Life was exciting, and incredibly busy. We did everything ourselves. It was a huge learning curve. We knew nothing about buying paper, finding good repro houses to scan in pictures and make the film, printing, distribution or selling advertising space. We learned from our mistakes, and some of them were very costly. But through it all came a steady stream of letters from readers, thanking us for their new-found confidence and self-esteem; wishing we had been around 20 years ago, before yo-yo dieting caused them to be much larger now than they were before they'd started on the diet treadmill.

We began to have an effect on the fashion market too. For our very first shoot there were perhaps five or six companies to supply plus size samples. But gradually the industry began to sit up and take notice. Ann Harvey launched at about the same time *YES!* did, then came Elvi, Richards AS, Sixteen47, Etam Plus and Rogers + Rogers. Marks & Spencer increased their size range and even did a bra offer with us. I found Anna Scholz at her degree show for St Martin's, featured her clothes and saw her company grow to success. Another young designer, Nicola Taffler, made some clothes for our funky, clubbing fashion shoot. Littlewoods saw the feature, and gave Nicola and her company And Y Not two pages in their home shopping catalogue. We produced some pretty ground-breaking stuff: running alongside the fashion which never preached about 'disguising' or 'slimming styles', there were many hard-hitting features, about the diet industry, prejudice and all the many issues around size. We supported barrister Helen Jackson in her campaign to change the law and make size prejudice in the workplace illegal and ran features by many talented contributors, men as well as women.

All the time we were pushing the boundaries out, little by little, towards size acceptance. In order not to 'frighten the horses' I felt the best way forward was to make people think and present them with reasonable argument for change. We never subscribed to the Fat and Proud movement, believing instead that size, in an ideal world, should be quite simply irrelevant, although to try and achieve that goal we did have to bang on about it quite a lot! I desperately wanted women to stop putting their lives on hold until that mythical day in the future when they might magically become size 12. With my experience of the fashion industry I knew that there was no point in campaigning to have wonderful clothes on offer if women did not then have the confidence to buy and enjoy wearing them. I wanted to give them the belief that they had the right to spend money on their appearance and to look and feel good right now, whatever size they were. It didn't seem such an impossible thing to ask.

YES! never did break even, and eventually ended up costing us a great deal of money, but you don't expect to make a profit in the first three years of trading, and I was working for something I believed in with all my heart and soul. We had problems with WH Smith, who began to discriminate against 'specialist' publications. People expected to find us in Smith's, so when we didn't appear on their shelves they presumed we had stopped publishing. Then came the coup de grâce: because of our distribution problems, we realised we needed to look for alternative outlets, and had been talking to Evans over three years, trying to persuade them to sell our magazine, as they had done with *Extra Special*. Eventually they agreed, and sold three issues over six months in selected stores, before telling us that they had been planning their own magazine all along. *Encore* launched in the autumn of 1996 and in my heart I knew it would mean the end for *YES!*. We couldn't hope to compete against a magazine with a huge company and so much money behind it that it was being given away free to many thousands of Evans budget card holders, and sold in-store for just £1, but we soldiered on.

Our sales slumped to less than half over the next year. Our advertising revenue was down, too, at an all time low, due I believe not only to our drop in circulation but also to the difficulties experienced by the small specialist shops, our mainstay, who were having their own bad time on the high streets – another case of Goliath beating up David. We could never get ads from the major fashion stores and catalogues or the make-up and perfume ads that support most glossy magazines. Large women are simply not perceived as being the right market for these precious products, although no doubt the manufacturers are willing enough to take our money. With barely any revenue coming in we searched around for an injection of capital, and talked to all the big publishing companies, trying vainly to find someone who believed in the project and its potential as much as we did, to no avail. We had to admit defeat in March 1998. After nearly five years we could no longer continue to publish and were forced to put our company into voluntary liquidation. We did eventually sell the title so that it would survive for the sake of our subscribers, and to cover at least part of what we owed to the bank. It almost broke my heart – at the time it felt as if I was giving up my baby for adoption. Unfortunately a sudden change in circumstances and the unexpected death of a major backer meant the relaunch of *YES!* has been put on ice, and the publishing company that bought it has no definite plans for its reappearance.

In those last few sad weeks we had dozens of calls from readers, asking where the next issue was, and expressing deep regret and support when told that we were unable to carry on. I realised that it had not all been for nothing. Success cannot only be measured in financial terms: there were many women who had felt uplifted and empowered by *YES!*. They at least had taken on board the message that life is for living now, and that so much effort is wasted in the pursuit of the perfect body. But there simply were not enough of them. The slimming magazines continue to flourish; Rosemary Conley still produces a new book every year; dieting is the only industry that is based on failure. In his book, *Ways of Seeing*, designer John Berger says of the effect advertising has on a woman: 'The publicity image steals her love of herself as she is, and offers it back to her for the price of the product.' Twenty-seven years on from when he wrote those profound words, British women are still buying into the myth. Yet research in America proves that 94% of people who lose weight through dieting put it all back on again, plus more, within five years. We know now that regular exercise and a healthy lifestyle are the keys, whatever your size; but unless or until we can also begin to value ourselves for the human beings we are – successful career women, wonderful mothers, caring partners, creative cooks, brilliant managers – for all the diverse roles we play, rather than worrying constantly about the way we look, whether we can pinch an inch, nothing can ever really change.

After a lifetime of banging my head against this particular brick wall which encloses us all, fat, thin or 'average', and undermines our potential as human beings so severely, am I to conclude that we have made no progress and that I have wasted my career achieving nothing, being nothing but a voice crying in the wilderness? No, of course not. You only have to read the other contributions in this book to understand how far we have come. I now have a part-time job as a lecturer in journalism, and am thrilled by my students' universal condemnation of prejudice in all its evil manifestations. I know many young, big women who are questioning the kind of treatment my generation has taken as the norm, and who will not accept second-class citizenship: one of them laughs out at me triumphantly from a huge poster whenever I pass the window of my local Body Shop. It is up to them to take over the torch and keep it burning brightly. As editor of *YES!* I helped many students who were tackling the complicated issues around size: fashion designers, photographers, aspiring journalists, young lawyers, film-makers; all of whom, as they emerge into womanhood and begin to enter the workforce, will start demanding equal treatment alongside their slimmer sisters. Then at last, not just the individual battles, for more fashion choices, for equal opportunities in employment, to be treated seriously – but the entire war, waged so that people of all shapes and sizes can live together without judgement or prejudice, will finally be won.

Confessions of a Failed Dieter

Sherry Ashworth

When I was nine, I was unpopular at school. I didn't have to wonder too long why this was so; my adversaries were keen to point out the reasons. They followed me home from school calling 'four eyes' and 'fattie'. This went on for a few months, until I confessed to my dad. Beat 'em up, he said. So one afternoon I attacked the ringleader, in a sixties version of Girl Power. I was hauled into school and branded as a Juvenile Delinquent, my parents tried to justify my actions, and the taunting mysteriously stopped.

By the time I was 12, my long-sightedness had corrected itself, and I was able to consign my specs to the dust heap. Four eyes was a thing of the past. Anyway, the taunt never really bothered me. I always knew I could take off my glasses whenever I wanted to. The fat, however, was a different affair.

Puppy fat, my mother called it. It'll soon go. I was determined to help it on its way. At 14 I experimented with eye-liner, blue eye shadow, and dieting. The latter consisted of eating as little as possible until about four o'clock when I couldn't stand the hunger any more. As I matured, I was able not to eat too much from Monday until Thursday, then I broke.

I still believe that had I not joined Weight Watchers, my dieting experiments would have been abandoned along with my roll-on pantie girdle and wet-look mini skirt. That was not to be. Weight Watchers started a group in the Loyola Hall in South Tottenham, and Aunty Sylvie offered to take me. I have to point out that Aunty Sylvie is not the villain of the piece.

She, and my mother, wanted me to be happy. If it was slimness I coveted, then they genuinely believed that by helping me to be slim, they would be making me happy. The orthodoxy of the time was that dieting was good for women.

And so I went to the Loyola Hall and sat rapt with attention as a petite forty-something in a smart suit preached to us about the joys of slimness and how easy it was to attain. She warned us against the demon double chocolate gateau with old adages such as, a moment on your lips, forever on your hips. Fattening food was *sinful*. Our bible was the Weight Watchers diet, which was so complex as to require a whole booklet and a good hour's study before it could be understood. New members had to stay behind to go over it.

From the moment our lecturer opened her mouth, I was hooked. Here was a new religion, with rules and rewards – our lecturer *was* the way, the truth and the life. Salvation was attainable with only two slices of bread a day and weighing your fruit – you must always weigh your fruit. Here, in the Loyola Hall, was another place to shine. I was a high achiever at school, and loved winning glittering prizes. At Weight Watchers too, I knew I could be a star.

I became passionate about my diet. Early Christian martyrs had nothing on me – I majored in mortification of the flesh. I forced myself to eat one liver meal a week, which I hated. I gagged as I ate it. I drank only Marvel skimmed milk and learned to love rhubarb – bowls and bowls of boiled rhubarb with artificial sweetener. And my weight began to plummet.

Dieting was an exquisite agony. I remember very clearly being invited to the bar mitzvah of an affluent school friend's brother at the Savoy Hotel. I stuck to my diet (!!!!). Eventually I hit a 'plateau'. This was Weight Watchers terminology for when your body is resisting the loss of any more weight. I found the plateau discouraging, but I soldiered on. The dieting was my proving ground. It was intimate, personal, and by withholding pleasure from myself, I was sure I was doing something good.

This is not going to be one of those stories when the young person in question descends into anorexia or bulimia. I don't know what it was that saved me from an eating disorder, as the causes of eating disorders can be so various, but in the end I couldn't stand the deprivation any more. I began to eat again. I never reached my goal weight at Weight Watchers (which was set impossibly and unhealthily low) and, feeling a failure, I gave up.

And I put the weight back on. Only slowly – I wasn't a binge eater. By the time I went to Oxford I was nicely rounded again. It made me feel that I ought to do something about it. Only it was tough; I was living away from home for the first time, and eating was comforting. I tried to push myself into dieting again by overeating – only an ex-dieter will understand the logic here. If you overeat like mad, than you've *got* to go on a diet. Stands to reason, mate. So I'd buy a stash of chocolate and open my Mars bar and copy of *Our Mutual Friend* simultaneously.

I think it was around this time that the dieting/overeating syndrome began to be a sort of displacement activity for me. If things were bad, they would come right again if I dieted. If things were bad, I could eat, and they would seem better. Either way I won, and both ways I lost. My fat became a visible symbol of all the things I didn't like about myself. Dieting – or, more often, thinking about dieting – gave me the illusion that I could change myself fundamentally. My low self-esteem located itself in my fat; because I was fat, I had low self-esteem.

But no shortage of boyfriends. I thought it paradoxical that boys I knew never focused on my size – except one, and I dropped him. My self-esteem wasn't *that* low. I can honestly say that no one important in my life has ever made me feel bad about my weight. I perpetrated my own ego-bashing.

In my early twenties, I hit the slimming club circuit again. Thinking Weight Watchers wouldn't have me back (as if!), I joined the now defunct Silhouette. We stood up at meetings and (this is true) recited together:

I must, I must, I must improve my bust!
I will, I will, I'll make it better still!
Hoorah! Hoorah! I need another bra!

I was 23, I was reading for a BPhil in Mediaeval Studies at the University of York, and I was reciting this, and believing it...

At 25 I married Brian, who was and still is utterly bemused at my preoccupation with my weight. I remember wishing I was slimmer on my wedding day, and thinking that one fine day, who knows?

Then I started teaching. As any new recruit to the classroom will tell you, being a probationary teacher is one of the most gruelling, exhausting activities ever devised for womankind. I began to eat again. Not only that, being married meant I was cooking more – and eating the results. I put on more weight than ever, and became wildly distressed. I had nightmares about getting fatter and fatter. I was actually scared of what I was becoming.

I went to the doctor. The doctor recommended yet another slimming group, this one run by a psychologist at a local hospital. He gave us a diet sheet and a regime of behavioural science. I lost weight. Once again, I liked losing more weight than anyone in the group. I discovered how easy it was to eat hardly anything at all. The kids at school complimented me on my weight loss. I wore tight jeans and was a size 12.

At last I'd got there. I was slim. But something was bothering me. I went back to the psychologist, a taciturn man with a ginger beard. I told him I was slim now, but I wasn't happy. I'd always imagined that when I was slim, I would enter a brave new world. The sun would shine perpetually, and every day would be the first day of spring. I asked him why I was now unhappier than ever, terrified of losing my new-found slimness, still not satisfied with the way I looked, hoping to lose just a pound or two more, to be on the safe side. Why? He said nothing, but looked baffled.

Slowly I put the weight back on again, and then I became pregnant with my first daughter. Bliss. I could put on weight and it was socially acceptable. I revelled in my pregnancy. I decided to try the Earth Mother hat on for size. I gave up work, stayed at home, breast-fed and changed nappies.

For me, a big mistake. I became quite depressed, and when we ran out of money soon after the birth of our second daughter, and I *had* to go back to work, I was overjoyed. And then I took stock. You've guessed it – I thought I needed to go on a diet. I messed around with the F-Plan (who didn't?) and tried just cutting back. Then the mother of a pupil suggested I go to Weight Watchers with her. I was 36. Why not, I said.

Only this time, twenty years on, it was different. I noticed things I hadn't noticed the first time round. How come all the new members were actually re-joiners? Hadn't the diet worked the first time? Why were there pictures of food everywhere in the meeting room? Why were we talking about food all the time when surely it would be more sensible to forget about food? Why were Weight Watchers and Heinz the same firm? Why was the lecturer confessing to her binges in front of us? What was an intelligent woman like me doing listening to this claptrap? Why, if I despised it all, was I still dieting?

I lost some weight, then it was Christmas, and I gave up. I thought, there has to be something better to do with my life than dieting. I decided it would be fun to try writing. I've always had the highest regard for writers, and have swooned at the feet of Doris Lessing, Salman Rushdie *et al.* It was precisely this high regard that stopped me writing. What was the likes of me doing, thinking she could be like the likes of them? Me – a fat person – what a cheek! But giving up dieting was a liberating time. It opened up new possibilities. It meant I could stop living conditionally (when I lose weight) and actually start living.

I began to keep a commonplace book filled with jottings, and showed it to a writer friend. He read it through and commented favourably on a description I'd written of a big woman I'd observed on the beach. I realised that weight was still an issue with me, and that I had accidentally become an expert in how not to deal with it. Thus the idea for my first novel, *A Matter of Fat*, was born.

I wanted it to be a comic novel because instinctively I felt that part of the answer to an obsession with weight was not to take oneself too seriously. It was a relief for me to expose, through fiction, the crazy dieting behaviour to which I'd become addicted. I wrote of how I'd binge on coming home from a slimming club meeting, confident the binge wouldn't show up on the scales next week, or how I'd weigh myself three or four times a day. I wrote of my own difficulties in adjusting to being a woman who wasn't going to diet again, making one character say that she would be perfectly happy to be a fat woman, if only she could be a few pounds slimmer. I think that sums it all up.

The best thing about *A Matter of Fat*'s success was that so many women identified with the behaviour I'd described in it. That was a revelation to me; I genuinely thought I was alone with my neurosis. Of course I'd read *Fat is a Feminist Issue*, but that only served to convince me I was fat *because* I was neurotic. I'm afraid that sanity seemed even further away than slimness. No one, but no one, has perfect parents, and I didn't want to blame my loving mother and father for my obsession with size. That's victim think. In my case, being neurotic had not made me fat; dieting had made me both neurotic *and* fat.

I always imagined that if my first novel was a success, I would magically grow up and care no more about being big. For a while, in the euphoria of having the novel published, this was true. What authority would I have as the creator of a comic novel slamming the diet industry, if I was slim? It was almost as good as being pregnant. I had an excuse to look the way I did.

Then reality kicked in. I learned that one couldn't overthrow a lifetime of dieting behaviour just like that. The most interesting part of my journey towards size acceptance began after I started to write about the issue.

Firstly, don't you believe anyone who tells you that they were able to make a sudden transformation from being weight obsessed to being anxiety free. Learning self-acceptance is a gradual process. Finding success as a novelist wasn't as helpful as one might imagine. I always felt that the pseudo-glam me at launches and author events was an actress; the real, still rather fat me, was the true Sherry.

The most important thing for me in learning to be large, has been the support of other large women. This is invaluable, even essential. In the beginning, I didn't think I looked very good, but it was easy for me to see that the other large women I knew *did* look good. Admiring other fat women made me see myself differently. I have to confess that I like to look good. I spend an embarrassingly large amount of money on cosmetics and relish applying make-up. I can't think for a moment that appearance doesn't matter. On giving up dieting, I had to learn a whole new way of presenting myself. That's been one of the most enjoyable parts of the process of size acceptance.

The next thing that's been instrumental in helping me be a happy size 20 has been the explosion of plus size clothes stores. Shopping has become a blissful experience. I can try on all sorts of clothes and only buy the ones that suit me, rather than the ones that fit. The temptation to diet to get into nice clothes is a thing of the past.

These days I observe myself carefully. I've noticed that when I'm stressed or depressed, I want to comfort eat *and* I simultaneously feel fat. When things are going well, I feel good about myself, and become less conscious of the place of food in my life. I can see more clearly how fat, for me, is a solid metaphor for my psychological state. Understanding this helps me to distance myself from a preoccupation with weight. I can unravel my own mind games. Knowledge is power.

What hasn't helped me come to terms with myself? Most prominently, society's new obsession with so-called 'healthy eating'. This is a tabloid age of crude moral certainties, and one of these is that Health is a Good Thing. We hear it argued that it can't be okay to be fat because it's unhealthy. What you look like is now conceded grudgingly to be a matter of choice, but health isn't. The NHS has only so many resources, and fat people tend to get ill. So do those who engage in dangerous sports, smokers, people who go to work in crowded trains and catch flu, people who work too hard, get stressed and weaken their immune systems – but none of these get the constant ridicule and insidious rejections that fat people suffer. I've noticed that among my friends those that seem to take the most time off work through ill health are the fittest – they're always straining their backs at the gym and pulling ligaments whilst jogging. Plump, sedentary people like me seem to enjoy enviable health. Fattism is highly illogical and utterly unjust.

And then there's so-called healthy eating. Everyone is expected to do this. Yet healthy eating is only another word for dieting. Just as downsizing replaced redundancy, healthy eating has replaced the dieting word. So everywhere we go we are met by diets masquerading as eating plans, and women are still being encouraged to relinquish control of their own bodies to some nameless authority who apparently knows better. Few experts are prepared to concede that *real* healthy eating should be natural, joyful, include reasonable amounts of chocolate and celebratory meals, be neurosis-free and that any form of consistent under-eating will take its eventual toll. As it did with me.

It's a cliché now that images of women affect the way we see ourselves, but like all clichés, it's true. I get dispirited after watching countless slim women on television. The effect it still has on me is to make me feel that in some subtle way, I don't fit. My body, a living history of yo-yo dieting and a couple of pregnancies, is the sort of body, I discover, that one really ought to keep under wraps. So I still feel uneasy about my appearance unless I wear trousers, long skirts, and tops with sleeves. Or perhaps this is just modesty – I hope so!

There's no doubt that I worry much less about weight these

days. Back in my twenties, I was either on a diet (starving) or off a diet (bingeing). I couldn't imagine life in the middle. Now, these pendulum swings are far less extreme. I go through phases of trying to cut down what I eat, and then I go through phases of not giving a toss.

The most compelling reason I have not to diet now is my two teenage daughters. The elder is the same age I was when I started my career as a Weight Watcher. Both of my daughters have the same body shape I did at their age. They are rounded, and both very pretty. The younger one enjoys sport, thanks to the new breed of games teacher who encourages rather than humiliates. Thanks, Miss Hill, Mrs Riley and Mrs Ferrol!

Both my girls enjoy food. Every so often I screw up and get them to join in my occasional binges, and I regret it afterwards. When I cut back, they copy me. I've learned a mother has an awesome influence on her daughters. This knowledge guides my behaviour around food, and stops me bad-mouthing myself if I don't like the way I look.

My daughters seem reasonably comfortable with themselves at present, and have swallowed whole my anti-dieting and anti-fattism philosophy, often sounding off about it over the school canteen dinner table. They like occupying the moral high ground! I feel fairly certain now that they won't be fodder for the dieting industry, and they won't torture themselves with feelings of not fitting in, of looking wrong, of there being too much of them.

I'm 45 now, and the good news is that the older you get, the less you worry about size. This is partly because you lose the self-centredness of youth, and get to see that other people are just as important as you, and often more so. The self-absorption of dieting behaviour seems unattractive. A good relationship with another person or with yourself is far more valuable than a good figure. On the other hand, the pain I inflicted on myself through my weight obsession has given me an insight into how to deal with different sorts of self-inflicted pain. Also I feel I have some empathy with others who feel excluded from mainstream society, as I did. These are precious gifts.

I also know there's a point where you realise you are who you are – and you can change your underclothes, but not your true self.

Both my maternal and paternal grandmothers were large women. They were also loving, hard-working, respected women. My mother is large. She's also gorgeous. I want to be like them, just as my daughters seem to want to be like me.

How We Met

An interview by Anthi Charalambous

Dawn French and Helen Teague

DAWN FRENCH

It was early 1990 and I was in search of good clothes, and I'd read about a shop called Big Clothes. On the day I went along, Helen's partner was there. I was buying loads of stuff, doing that panic-buying that big women do when they finally come across reasonable clothes.

I could hear Helen downstairs, working on her sewing machine. Then it stopped and she came up. She looked at me and said: 'I've been waiting for you to come here.' Helen is very spiritual and thinks that it was fate that I walked through the door. For a second I wondered: 'Do you know me?'

She seemed slightly mysterious to me. I was struck by how beautiful she was, with this big open face and huge smile that completely lit it up. I remember trusting her straight away. She was quite a big girl and wearing great clothes – this bodes well, I thought. Helen was immediately very honest and advised me to reconsider several of the choices I'd made. I liked her directness – she wasn't at all in awe of me.

About a year later she came to see me in the play *Silly Cow* and afterwards came backstage to my dressing-room and pitched the whole partnership idea to me. I'd been thinking of a similar venture for about a year and approached various designers to investigate how much it would cost. But it would have meant remortgaging the house and I'm too cautious to risk everything. So when Helen came along, she was the answer.

Our workshop is based in Ghana, and Helen spends part of the year there. I miss her when she's not here. We talk on the phone a lot and she sends me faxes and letters, occasionally touching on business matters. When all that is going well, which is most of the time, we toast ourselves with champagne.

We socialise together a lot. We quite quickly got intimate about personal things, and both relish a good gossip. I often invite Helen to parties – she was at my 40th. We're members of a small secret society, the Lazy Sues, five girls and one 'honorary' who take regular singles holidays together. We set out to have fun and we do – there's quite a lot of nail-painting involved.

Helen's also part of the book club that Jennifer [Saunders] and I started. If there is a consensus about a book, Helen will differ, not because she's contrary but because she has such a quirky view of life. The wiring in her head is connected in a different way from other people's.

Helen knows all my secrets and has seen the worst side of me, and doesn't mind. I get grumpy when I'm anxious and under pressure. I know she would never badmouth me, and among my women friends that kind of loyalty is rare.

I find her astute observations of the people we both know very intriguing. Helen's judgement on work matters is excellent, though in her personal life it's more questionable. I'd like to matchmake for her, although I think she's perfectly capable of doing it for herself. But her advice across the board is always worth listening to. Helen possesses an ancient wisdom.

We're both certifiable workaholics. Helen is passionate about her work, so much so that she's sacrificed an awful lot for it – a family life of her own and a chunk of her social life. But it fulfils her – it's like great sex to her. She doesn't own anything, she lives like a student and has no interest in material things. Her priorities are different.

Helen is an eternal optimist – her glass is always half-full. I'll be surprised if she ever loses her enthusiasm. She once had a

God-is-it-worth-the-effort? turn and I was shocked. That's my role – hers is always to see the best in everything.

In lots of ways, Africa is her true home. When she moved back she felt much more comfortable – big women are celebrated over there. Helen spends a lot of time absolutely baffled by British culture. I didn't know Helen had African heritage to begin with, but she and Lenny clicked immediately – there was a great resonance between them.

I would like Helen to rate herself more highly – I'd like her to know in her heart what a good person she is. She's very intelligent, perceptive and well-read. It's taken me quite a long time to get to know her, and I feel there is a lot more to know, and I know that it's all good.

Helen is a fantastically talented, artistic, gracious humanitarian and an unsung hero of design, in my opinion. She's elegant and sensual. If the business finished, we'd still be chums because I need her to be in my life. I rely on her an awful lot now for her counsel. She'll never let me down. Helen is cheaper than a psychiatrist. I wouldn't want to be without her, that's for sure.

HELEN TEAGUE

Dawn walked into my shop at ten past five in the afternoon on 18 January 1990. I had a shop called Big Clothes in St John's Wood. I was in the tiny basement, cutting and stuff, and I heard this distinctive voice. I went upstairs and when my head was level with the floor, I looked up at her and said: 'Are you Dawn French? I've been waiting for you.' We'd been trading for two years and I knew she'd come. I remember writing in my diary that I sensed there was something fateful in the encounter.

I could tell that she was very shy. My partner kept pointing her in the direction of brighter stuff, and I sensed she wanted something more sophisticated. Dawn is wonderful on camera, but people tend to associate her with her screen characters. I never did – I realised that she was actually quite a serious person. I've never stood on ceremony with people; she came to my shop for a service, and she got it.

A year later, my business partner and I went our separate ways. I wrote to Dawn on impulse to ask whether she'd be interested in buying a share in our shop. I'd read somewhere that she had wanted to do something like this before, so it wasn't a complete shot in the dark.

The play *Silly Cow* was running and one evening I went backstage to broach the subject. She'd already made up her mind, it seemed. It was rather funny – we were soon chatting about children and all that personal stuff, and at the end of it all I wasn't sure whether she'd said yes or not. I asked, 'Are you up for this then?' and she said, 'Yeah, I'll give it a whirl.'

We're both extremely busy and have to snatch our time together. We never have enough time to sit around in companionable silence, being entertained in dark venues. We're too busy with salacious gossip. Dawn calls me regularly, but I prefer to write. I've got a mental block about phones, my flat is full of them – it's a telephone graveyard.

We formed a clique of friends when we became partners, and all got drunk over pina coladas at breakfast and christened ourselves the Lazy Sues. We take sunshine holidays together and have a lark. The book club is another shared ritual, and a great excuse for a boisterous get-together at Groucho's.

Dawn has a sideways view of people – all her friends are unusual. She doesn't have conventional taste in anything. She thinks I'm a bit of a crank – I'm quite involved with astrology – but when I'm out with her I look around me and think I'm in good company.

We're both very visual, into art and aesthetics. Dawn has a very well-developed sense of style that spills over into everything. Her home is impeccably furnished, and she has a love of beautiful fabrics. We're creatively compatible. I don't hesitate to buy her presents to wear and objects for the house, and vice versa.

Through joining forces with Dawn I've been exposed to a whole new world. We have rigorous discussions – not arguments – because we deal in a world that is complex and frustrating. Ours is a feisty relationship. To be a friend in my life, a person has to be honest and have integrity. I don't have time to play games.

Dawn works very hard. My theory is that actually she'd like to live dangerously, that she has a wild streak that she reins in. Dawn's not really a risk-taker and so one of her ways of living life on the edge is to cram in too much work.

We have common ethical values. It makes a big difference that she's married to an Afro-Caribbean. I like the fact that when I visit their home it's not all white. She's completely clued into racism, a difficult area, and I never have to explain.

Dawn is still shy and a very private person. At home she's a loving wife and mother and enjoys domesticity. But it doesn't surprise me that she's a star, she's brilliant in her work. She'd have made a wonderful and remarkable teacher though, because she still would have had an audience and would have made a huge impact on people's lives.

Fate has brought us together. We've grown together and are much more worldly than we were when we met. It shows in our appearance and outlook. We have so much in common that if we weren't doing fashion we'd be something else together. We have a great deal of affection for one another; I adore her and feel very protective towards her. Dawn is steadfast and holds on to her friends, and so do I. Dawn is part of the fabric of my life, she's a reference point for me. We'll be together till we're both pushing up daisies.

Contributors' Notes

Sherry Ashworth is an English teacher, freelance writer, reviewer and broadcaster as well as author of seven comic, issue-based novels including *A Matter of Fat* and *Just Good Friends. What's Your Problem?*, published in the Livewire series, is her first novel for teenagers. She has also written a non-fiction book for the same age group – *Fat* – helping those who are preoccupied with food and weight. She was born and brought up in north London, but moved to Manchester in the seventies, and lives there with her husband, two daughters, two cats and a permanent supply of Uncle Joe's Mint Balls. No one in her household diets, or is allowed to diet.

Janice Bhend is a journalist and broadcaster, who founded and edited *YES!* magazine for plus-size women in 1993. The glossy bi-monthly was published nationally for almost five years, and one of its coverlines – Style is an Attitude Not a Size – equally applies to Janice. As a large teenager, she started her career in magazines in the sixties when it was only acceptable to be Twiggy sized and has been writing and campaigning ever since for more fashion choices and a better deal for larger women. Her ambition is to continue to combat stereotyping and discrimination in all its unpleasant manifestations. 'People should understand', she says, 'that it's not how we look but who and what we are that is important in life. So much human potential is wasted through senseless prejudice.' She believes that *YES!* did indeed change attitudes and help to empower a new generation of big, confident, unapologetic women. As a freelance she has contributed to national magazines and books and appeared on numerous radio and TV programmes over more than 20 years. She acts as a consultant on size matters to the media and is also a part-time lecturer in periodical journalism.

Jo Brand left her job as a psychiatric nurse in 1987, and since then has built up a large following on the London comedy circuit and throughout the UK. As Perrier Pick of the Fringe award nominee at the 1992 Edinburgh Festival and winner of the British Comedy Award for 'Best Live Performer' in 1992 and 1995, Jo Brand has been described by critics as 'The best female comic in Britain' (*Daily Mirror*). She has appeared widely on TV and radio, including her own show *Through the Cakehole*, 1993–5. She also currently writes a fortnightly column for the *Independent on Sunday*.

Jane Goddard Carter is an arts educated 38-year-old freelance film and television researcher, living in the West Country. She is fat. She has been fat for all of her life. She has experienced all the usual adversity that fat people have to deal with in their everyday lives. She honestly believes that if you are fat you have to deal with as much discrimination as any other minority group in this culture. It seems that to be openly hostile against fat people, particularly fat women is one of the last great allowable prejudices. After years of bowing to this nonsensical treatment, she finally had enough, and she now openly challenges it whenever and however she can. In the industry she works in, to be fat is often seen as an unacceptable state. The prejudice is sometimes unspoken, but is there none the less. Sometimes she believes she has to work doubly hard to secure jobs that could easily be given to younger, thinner people. Despite this, she lives happily, seeking out experiences to enrich her life and that of the world around her. She delights in the natural world and has an active interest in encouraging the humane treatment of all living things. This all sounds a bit sickly and rather like the blurb for a beauty contest, so she would like to add that she also goes like the clappers.

Dawn French studied at Central School. She was an original member of the Comic Strip, performing with her TV-partner-to-be Jennifer Saunders in the evenings while teaching drama during the day. She is married to Lenny Henry and they live in Berkshire with their daughter.

Ali Jacques has been described as 'an inspirational fat muse', and once, clad entirely in red sequins, was told by Jean Muir, 'You look marvellous, darling!' but never dared believe it! When she did, some years later, her column, 'Al's Mythbusters', set out to persuade readers of *YES!* magazine to 'throw away the sacks and brighten, not lighten your size 16, 28 or 48 shape!' From Central St Martin's to Comedy Nation, writer, actress, singer and artist – ignoring preconceived ideas that there are some things a fat girl shouldn't do – Ali set out to change media attitudes towards fat, because, she says, the concept of people openly enjoying their fat, and choosing to remain so, still baffles journalists! 'After pandering to other people's conditions for so long, I want to succeed by my own rules, and I'm a big girl with ambition to match my size, so look out!'

Stephanie Jones is a 38-year-old woman of African-Caribbean heritage. She has been involved in the UK size acceptance movement for many years. She currently works full-time as the co-ordinator of a health advocacy project for people living with HIV in Enfield, and has worked in the field of HIV for 12 years. Freelance training and management consultancy are part-time occupations, and Stephanie has worked with a large range of organisations. Singing is very close to Stephanie's heart, as she has sung since childhood, and has a mezzo-soprano voice with a rare four-to-five octave range. She also occasionally runs vocal training workshops. Stephanie sings in a wide variety of styles, but jazz is her favourite. Her most recent triumph was at the Victoria and Albert Museum, singing lead with the London Gospel Workshop. Nursing was Stephanie's original choice of career, and from there she moved on to gain several years' local government experience, followed by several more years in the voluntary sector. Along the way, she also trained as a counsellor and studied eating disorders. Stephanie has a keen interest in interior design, and is halfway through an interior-design course. She also recently commenced a management course. Stephanie is single (but likes to mingle!) and lives in North London with her two cats, Bibi and Mimi.

Angela Kennedy is a Researcher in the Gender Research Centre at Middlesex University. She is editor of an anthology *Swimming Against the Tide* published by Open Air Press in 1997. She has written for many publications, and is currently undertaking a PhD at Middlesex University on social constructions of fat women. She is married with a daughter, son, and a dog that needs a lot of walking. She plays the tin whistle, and since getting bigger, she swims like a fish!

Lee Kennedy, New York born artist, is a long-time denizen of the UK alternative cartoonist community. Her strips appear in numerous anthologies such as *Flock of Dreamers, Stripburger XXX, Women out of Line, What is This Thing Called Sex?* and she is a regular contributor to *Freesize*, the UK's size acceptance magazine. She also enjoys illustrating books such as Shelley Bovey's *Being Fat Is Not a Sin*, Avedon Carol's *Nudes, Prudes and Attitudes* and Vicky Barker's *Back on Top*. Her solo comic books, the *Inner City Pagan* and *Little Girl Blues* series, are available from Slab-O-Concrete, PO Box 148, Hove BN3 3DQ.

Miriam Margolyes is simply the most famous female voice in the UK. Known as 'the queen of the voice-overs', she started in radio in 1965 straight from Cambridge University and joined the BBC Drama Repertory Company, playing everything from old ladies to little boys, working with Paul Scofield, Sir Donald Wolfit, John Osborne, Coral Brown, Claire Bloom and honing the technique for which she has been called 'a radio actress of genius'. The invaluable experience of radio guided her into a career unrivalled in Britain for versatility and this range was given full scope in the thousands of TV and radio commercials she has broadcast since 1974 when her voice-over career took off. She was the voice for the entire British Royal Family in the runaway best-seller *The Queen And I*, now the most popular spoken-word cassette ever issued, for which she won the Sony Best Radio Actress 1993 Award. In 1997, Miriam was awarded the Best Performer in Audio Books for her recording of *The Portrait of a Lady* for the BBC. Her most recent TV roles in England are as the Head of Security in Lynda La Plante's *Supply and Demand* and as Miss Crawley in the classic BBC TV serial *Vanity Fair*. She has starred in her own sitcom *Frannie's Turn* on American TV and won the BAFTA Best Supporting Actress 1994 for her role in Martin Scorsese's film *The Age of Innocence* and was invited to join the American Academy. She starred in *James and the Giant Peach* as odious Aunt Sponge with Joanna Lumley as her sister, Spiker. In England she was last seen as Mrs Beetle in John Schlesinger's *Cold Comfort Farm*. She was the voice of Fly, the mother dog, in *Babe* and *Babe Two* and will be in the controversial, soon-to-be-released award-winning film about transsexuals, *Different For Girls*. She was nominated Best Supporting Actress by the London Film Critics for her Nurse in William Shakespeare's *Romeo and Juliet*. She has just filmed *The Taste of Sunshine* in Budapest with Ralph Fiennes and is about to star in *End of Days* with Arnold Schwarzenegger. Her last West End appearance, for which she received rave notices, was starring as George in *The Killing of Sister George* and she has also appeared in London in *Orpheus Descending* and *She Stoops to Conquer*, both for Sir Peter Hall.

Gladeana McMahon is a Fellow of the British Association for Counselling with a range of published material to her credit. She has more than twenty years' experience of helping people with a range of psychological difficulties. She is News Editor of *Counselling* and Managing Editor of *Stress News*. Apart from her many and varied professional activities, including a thriving psychotherapy practice, she is also heavily involved in the media, appearing on a range of television and radio programmes. She lives in South East London with Michael and their two cats and has a keen interest in enjoying life. She most recently started to learn to play the piano.

Maggie Millar was born in Australia and has worked in the entertainment industry for over thirty years. She toured Australia and New Zealand with Vivien Leigh and the Old Vic Company (a young Patrick Stewart was one of the actors). On going to London, she was awarded a scholarship to study at RADA (a young Anthony Hopkins was one of the students). She has appeared in many Australian television series including *The Sullivans* and *Prisoner, Cell Block H*, in the films *Phar Lap*, *Bushfire Moon* and *Pieta*, has worked extensively in theatre and radio and has won three awards for excellence for her work in theatre and television. She has been an active member of the Media and Entertainment Arts Alliance (formerly Actors' Equity), having served on the National Executive, and the Victorian Women's committee, which was concerned with the portrayal and status of women in the industry. She also served as the Public Relations Officer for Jigsaw Victoria, an organisation which successfully lobbied the Government for changes to adoption legislation. As a result of being a 'career dieter', for the past eight years she has conducted seminars, lectures and workshops for students, women's groups and health professionals on Body Image, Fat Phobia, Diet Myths and Self-Acceptance, and the total insanity of our obsession with what she calls 'physical correctness'. She lives with her husband in rural Victoria, where she can indulge her love of pastel painting, reading, listening to music and 'just looking out of the window'.

Jenni Murray has been the regular presenter of Radio 4's *Woman's Hour* since 1987. She also presents *Weekend Woman's Hour* each Saturday. She was born and educated in Barnsley, and has a degree in French and Drama from Hull University. Jenni joined BBC Radio Bristol in 1973. She went on to be a reporter and presenter for BBC TV's *South Today* in 1978, where she worked until 1983 when she joined *Newsnight*. She moved to Radio 4 in 1985 as a presenter for the *Today* programme and launched the Saturday edition of the programme with John Humphrys in 1987. Jenni is the author of *The Woman's Hour*, a history of women since World War II. She contributes to numerous newspapers and magazines and is an occasional documentary film-maker. She writes a weekly column in the *Express* each Tuesday. Jenni's interests include riding horses, the theatre, needlepoint and knitting and she is Vice President of the Family Planning Association. She has two sons.

Diana Pollard is a professional counsellor and size acceptance campaigner. She has a special interest in the way mental health professionals work with size and weight issues. She runs workshops and training courses on size acceptance and authentic living. Diana co-founded SIZE, the national size acceptance network: a forum of fat men and women committed to proactive lifestyles through personal empowerment, self-help and campaigning strategies. She co-edits *Freesize* magazine, a publication supporting the work of the British size acceptance movement. Diana's personal philosophy is also the byword of *Freesize* – 'Freedom to be the person you are'.

Esther D Rothblum is Professor of Psychology at the University of Vermont USA. She has co-edited 21 books, including *Overcoming Fear of Fat*, and her research has focused on the stigma of weight and on lesbian issues. She is editor of the *Journal of Lesbian Studies* and past editor of the journal *Women & Therapy*. Esther is a member of the Advisory Board of the National Association to Advance Fat Acceptance (NAAFA) and President of the Society for the Psychological Study of Gay, Lesbian, and Bisexual Issues of the American Psychological Association.

Joanne Simms fell asleep during a Latin lesson at the age of 14 and woke up two years later, to find herself sweeping the floor of the *Ashton Under Lyne Reporter*. She firmly believes she was very lucky to have had an old-fashioned, hot metal apprenticeship in journalism in the heady days before mobile phones, pagers, and laptops were invented, and no one ever dreamed of saying they worked 'in the meejia'. She is the news editor of *The Oban Times* group of newspapers in the West Highlands, because if you have to work for a living you might as well do so in the most beautiful place on earth. In 1998 she won the fourteenth *Mail on Sunday* novel competition and has just published her first novel, *Big Fibs and Little Fibs*.

Sally E Smith has spent a lifetime wrestling with weight issues. As a yo-yo dieter who was put on her first weight loss regime at the age of seven, Sally internalised the sense of failure and worthlessness that accompanies the cycles of weight loss and regain. In her late twenties, Sally decided that instead of trying to change the size of her body, it might be easier to change society's attitude about weight. To that end, Sally worked for 11 years as executive director of the National Association to Advance Fat Acceptance, an organisation dedicated to size acceptance advocacy, education and support. During that time, she staged demonstrations, lobbied for changes in public health policy about weight, and co-organised the Million Pound March. Now the editor-in-chief of *BBW* magazine – a fashion and lifestyle publication for plus-size women – Sally continues her work in the size acceptance movement, encouraging women to celebrate their beauty at any size. In addition, Sally has a son, Morgan, and is a Star Trek aficionado.

Kathryn Szrodecki has always been a fat London girl in a family that despises fat. Her first love was ballet, then school sports – so when the health club boom boomed in the early eighties, she joined her local club. Realising she was usually the only large woman in sight, she counted up the benefits she received from regular exercise and decided to qualify as an instructor. She passed her first YMCA qualification, exercise to music, in 1993 and started teaching, slowly building up her Greater Shape classes. In 1996 she produced the first fitness video for large women, again called *Great Shape*, and in 1998 she gained her YMCA Gym Instructor Award. She is currently opening her own health and fitness centre, which will be governed by a charter signed by all employees and freelancers guaranteeing no body discrimination – imagine, a chance to take your clothes off without judgement! In addition to this, Kathryn started a fashion business at age 19, and has gone on to transform it into Alternative Size – a mail order catalogue for large size clothing. She is also setting up a website called www.Larger.com, containing listings and news for larger people. She has a beloved, appreciative, supportive man in her life called Asher, and they are expecting their first child. They live in London with a cat, Boy-Boy, who also appreciates a wide lap.

Susan Stinson is the author of two novels and a book of poetry and short fiction. Passion for language and an abiding interest in the complex lives of fat women are central to her work. In addition to her novel-in-progress she is also working on a non-fiction project, *Too Much: Fat, Pleasure and Greed*. Her work has been featured in magazines including *Radiance*, *The Kenyon Review* and *Diva*, and in the video, *Gracious Flab/Gracious Bone*. She lives in Northampton, Massachusetts, near a river, low hills, and wonderful communities of friends, writers and fat activists.

Liz Swinden was born in Manchester in 1946. She trained as a teacher in Birmingham, taught for ten years in Sheffield and London then went to work for the NHS in 1985 supporting schools in developing Personal, Social and Health Education. She has written several publications for schools on sex education, drugs education and mental health. She helped organise the national Fat Women's Conference in 1989 and has been involved in size acceptance ever since. Her book for schools, *LifeSize*, co-written with Lesley de Meza, was published in 1999 by Forbes Publications. Her pleasures are singing in a women's choir, reading voraciously and tending her garden in Brighton, where she currently lives.

Helen Teague is a fashion designer. She trained as an architect while selling her clothes from a market stall. In 1986, she opened a shop in North London, and in 1991 she teamed up with Dawn French to launch another shop, Sixteen47, and their own label. Helen divides her time between Ghana, where her dogs Pluto and Pallas live, and England. Sixteen47 is at 69 Gloucester Avenue, London NW1 (0171 483 0733). French & Teague is also available in Evans outlets.

Betty Woods, artist/photographer, is the co-editor and designer of *Freesize* magazine. Betty graduated from Winchester School of Art in 1996 after completing a Fine Art Printmaking degree. Her work is mainly photographic/enhanced digital media and large screenprints. Betty believes that 'regardless of a person's body shape or size, the same basic human right should apply. "We" should not be segregated or penalised for such "offences". Fat is not a second-class label. It is a descriptive term, not a negative one. We should all stand up and fight to break down the barriers of ignorance. It may be difficult to swim against the tide, but to make progress, we have to re-evaluate how we feel about our own bodies before we can look through unbiased eyes and without prejudice.'